THE STORY OF CANCER
Volume 5

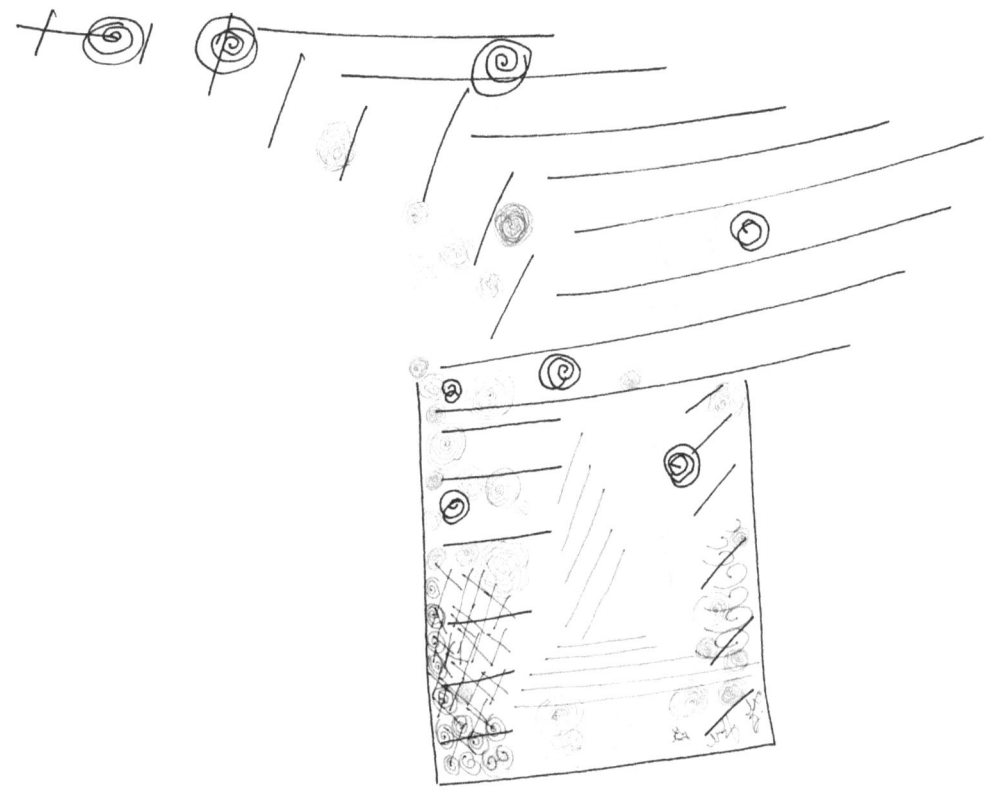

Camilia MacPherson, Ph.D., D.Th.
2016

INTRODUCTION

This is the Story of Cancer told using Automatic Drawings and Surreal Art. It is part of a continuous document written in 7 volumes.

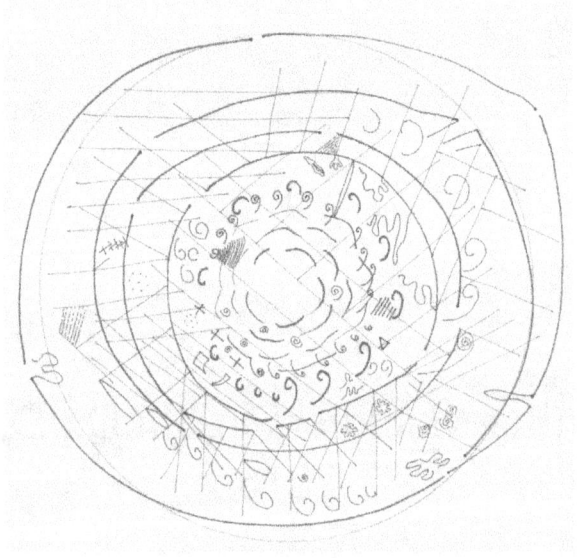

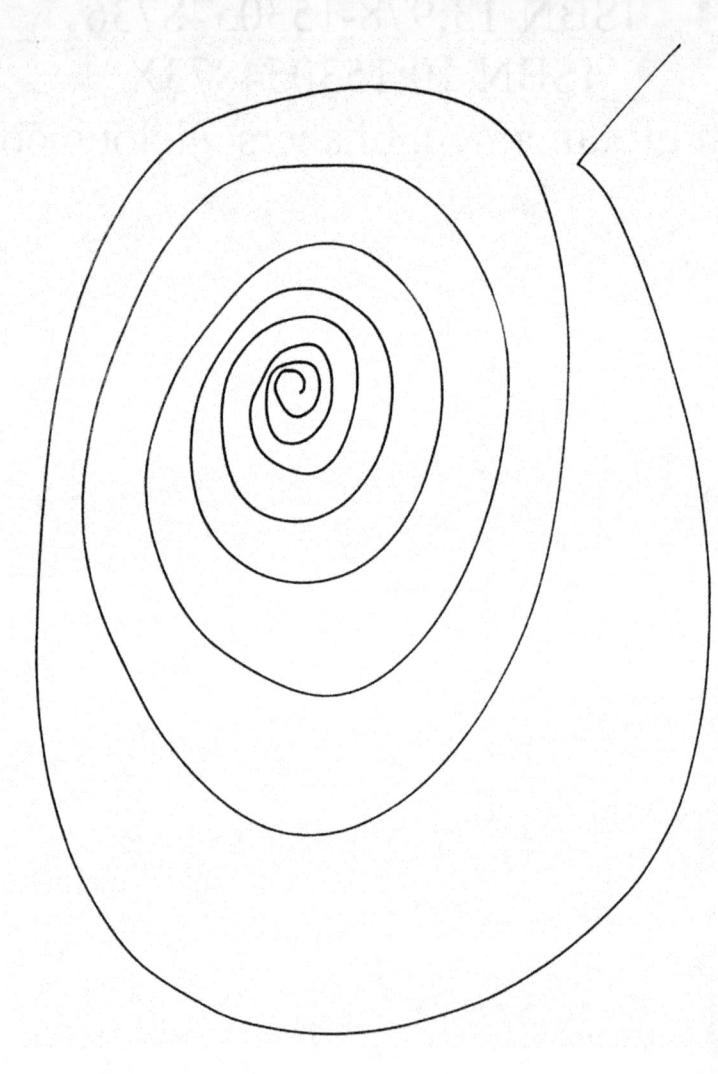

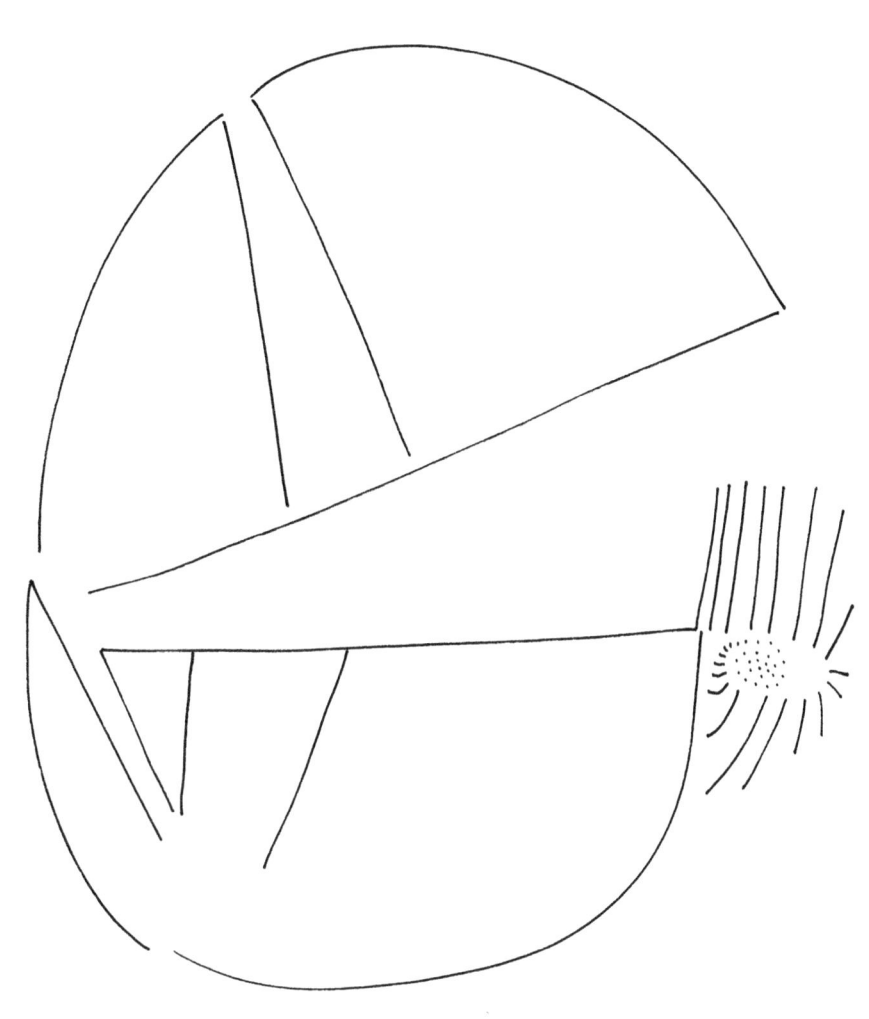

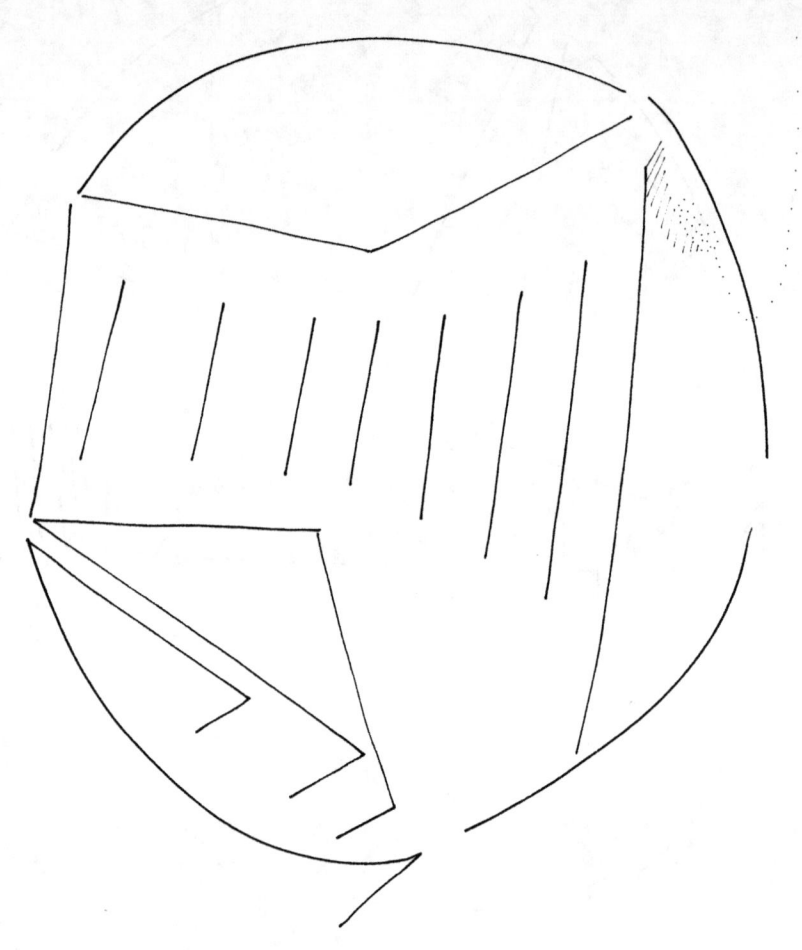

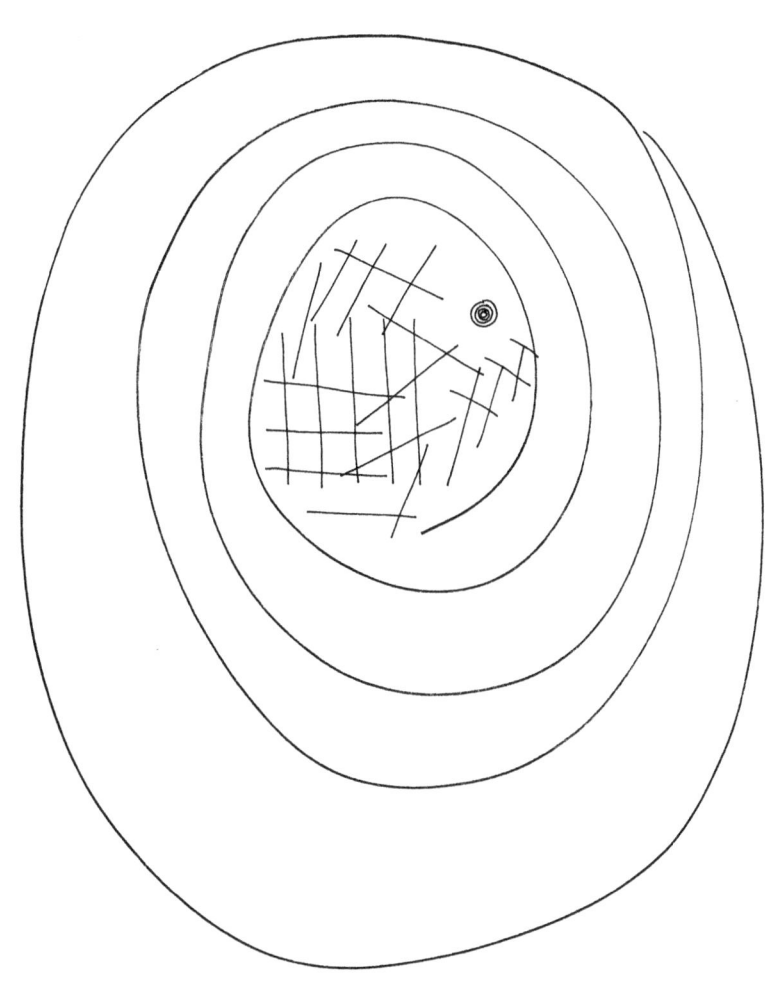

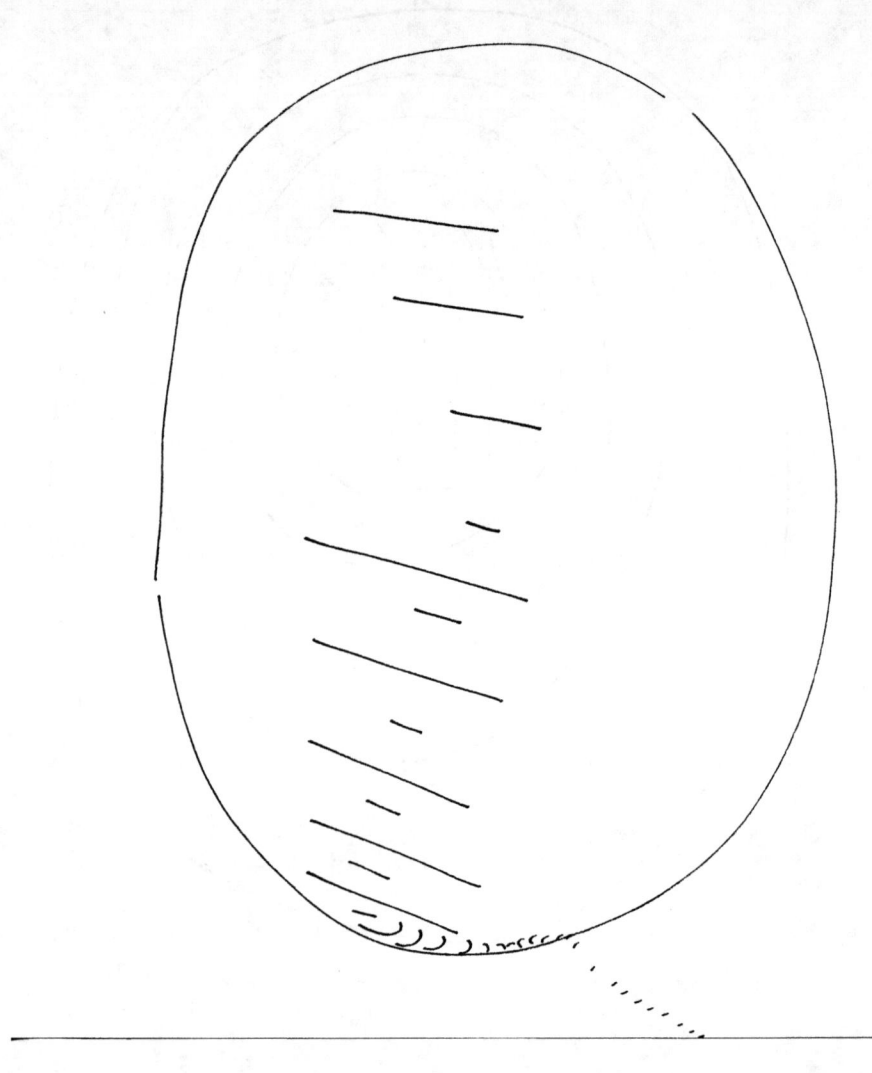

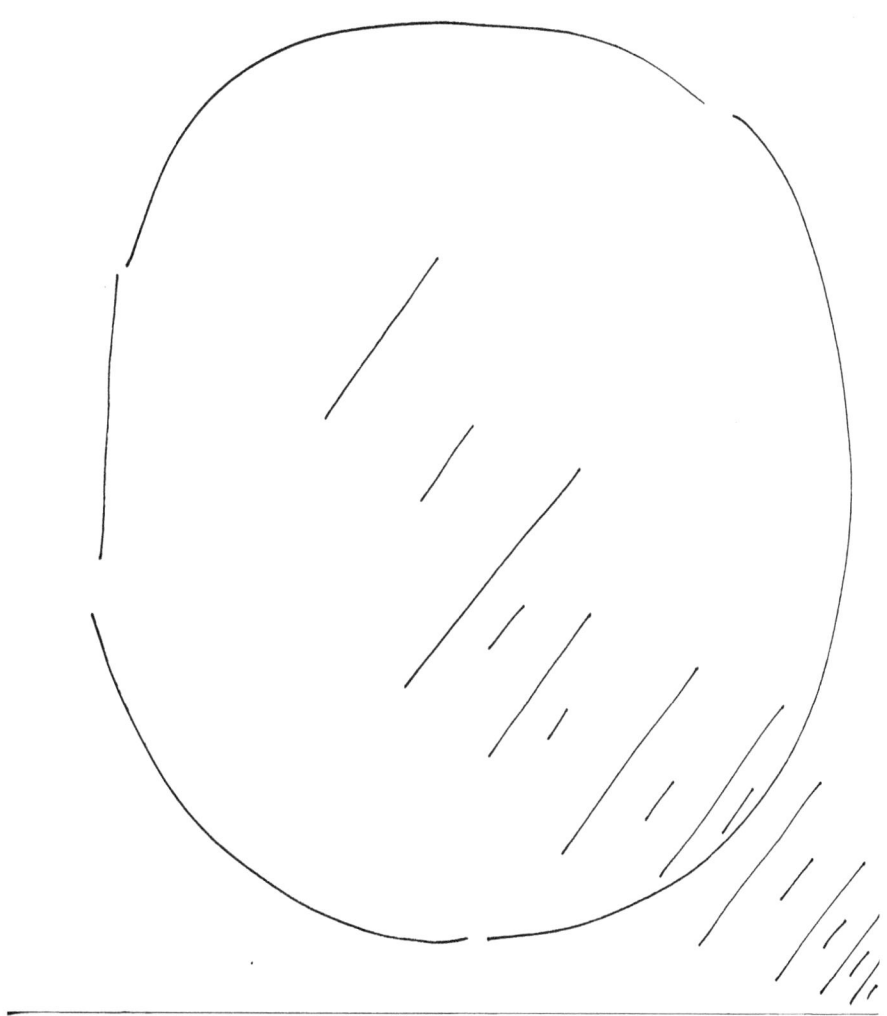

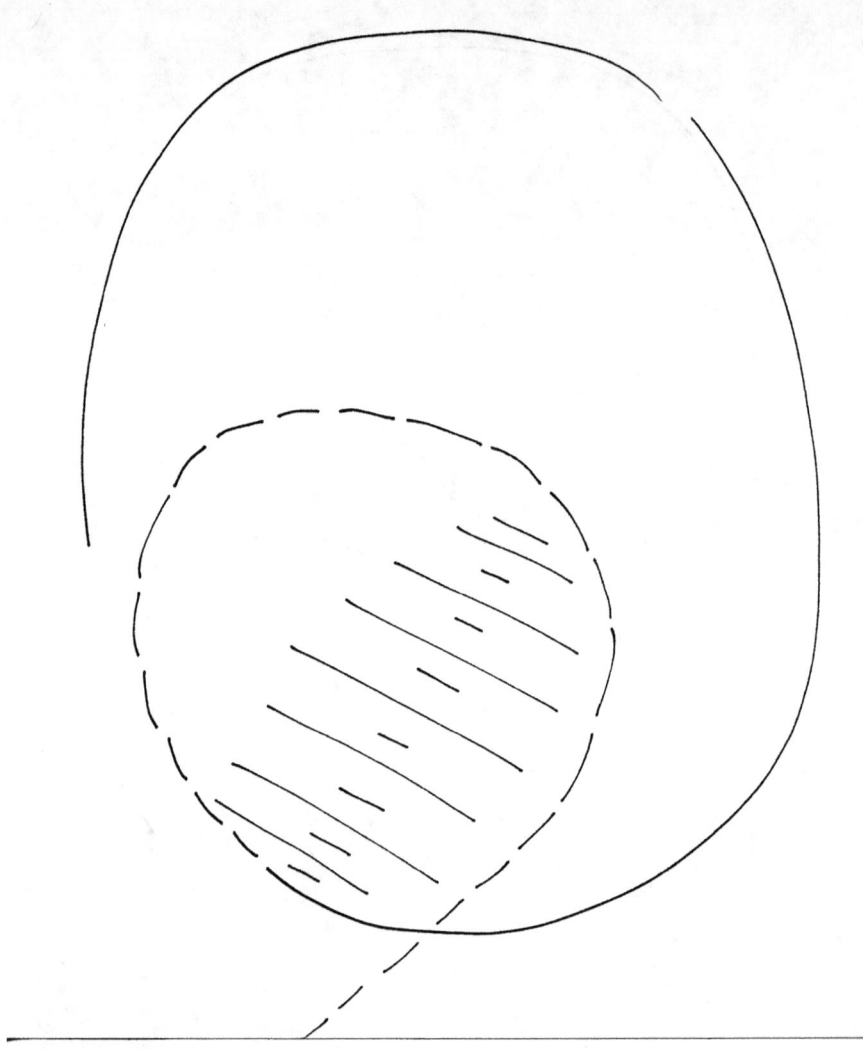

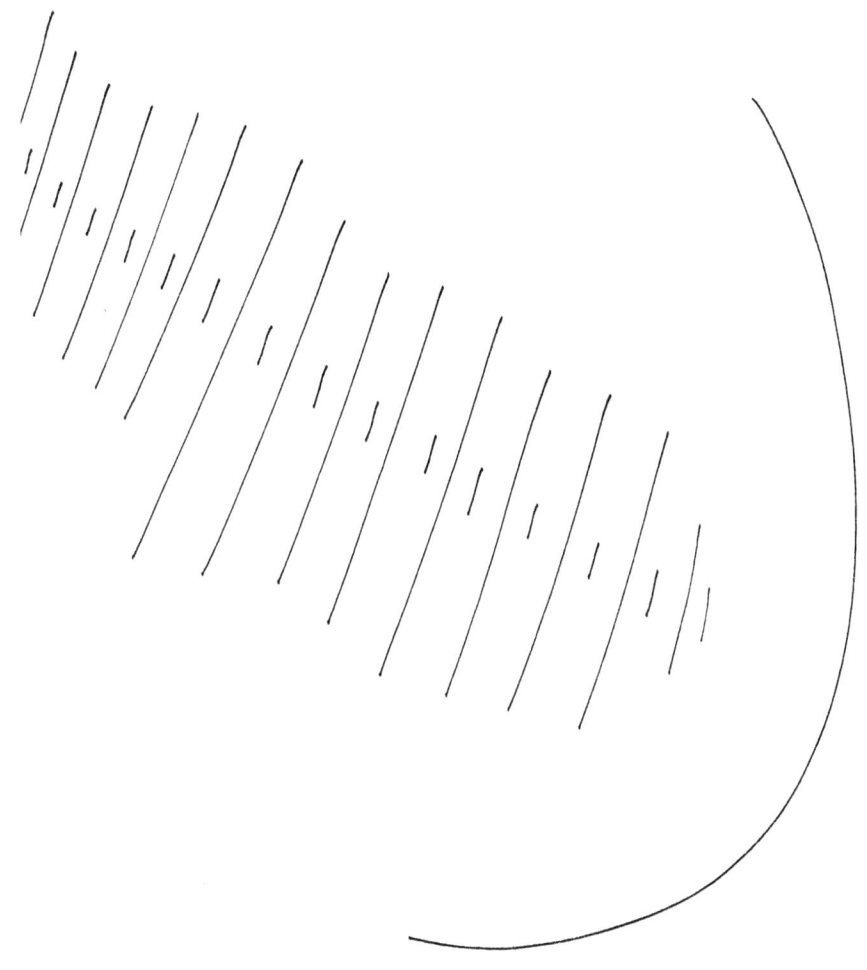

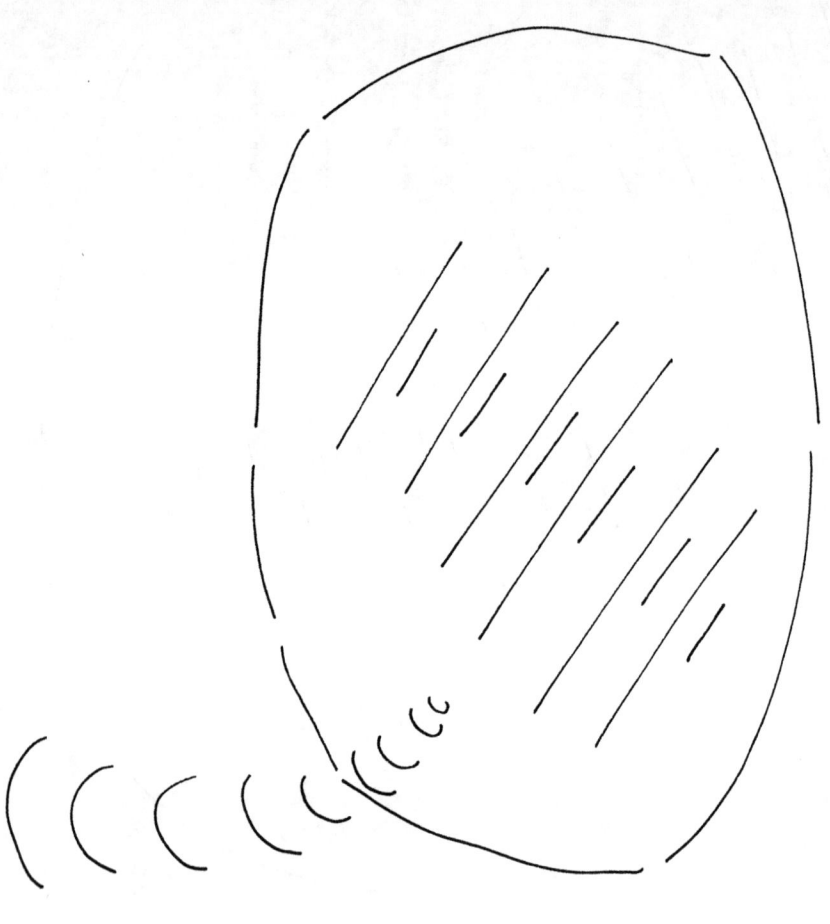

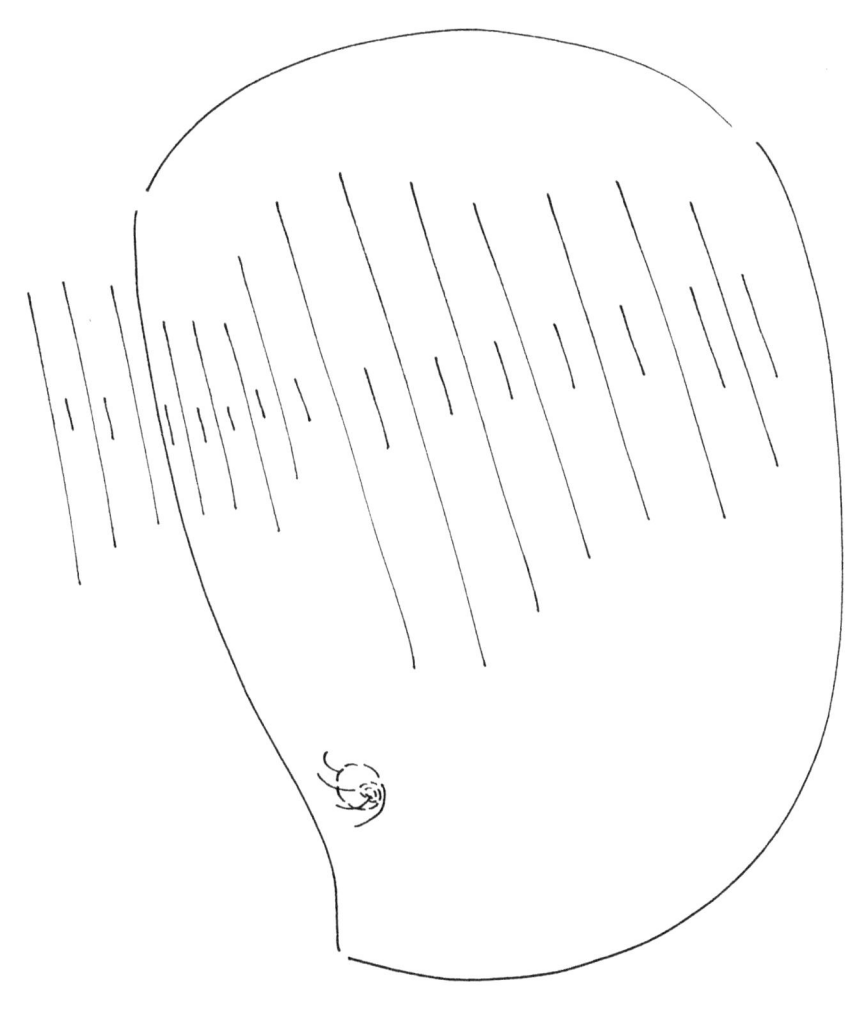

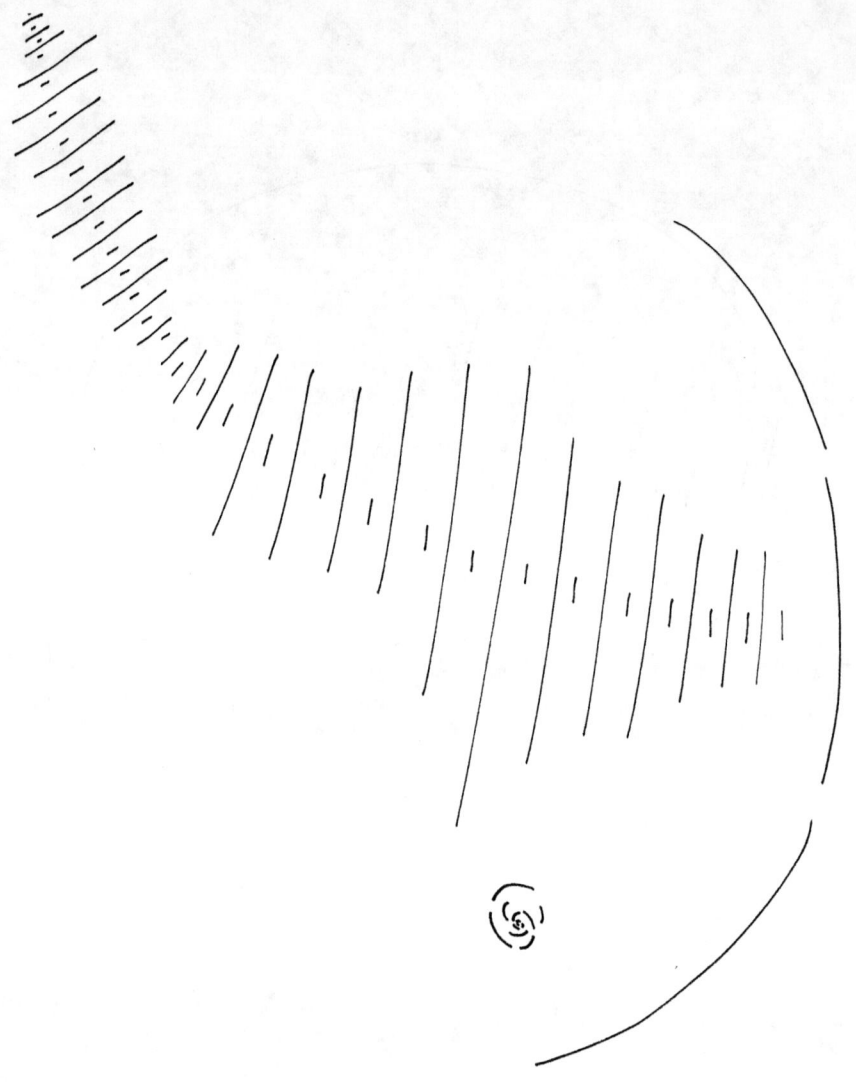

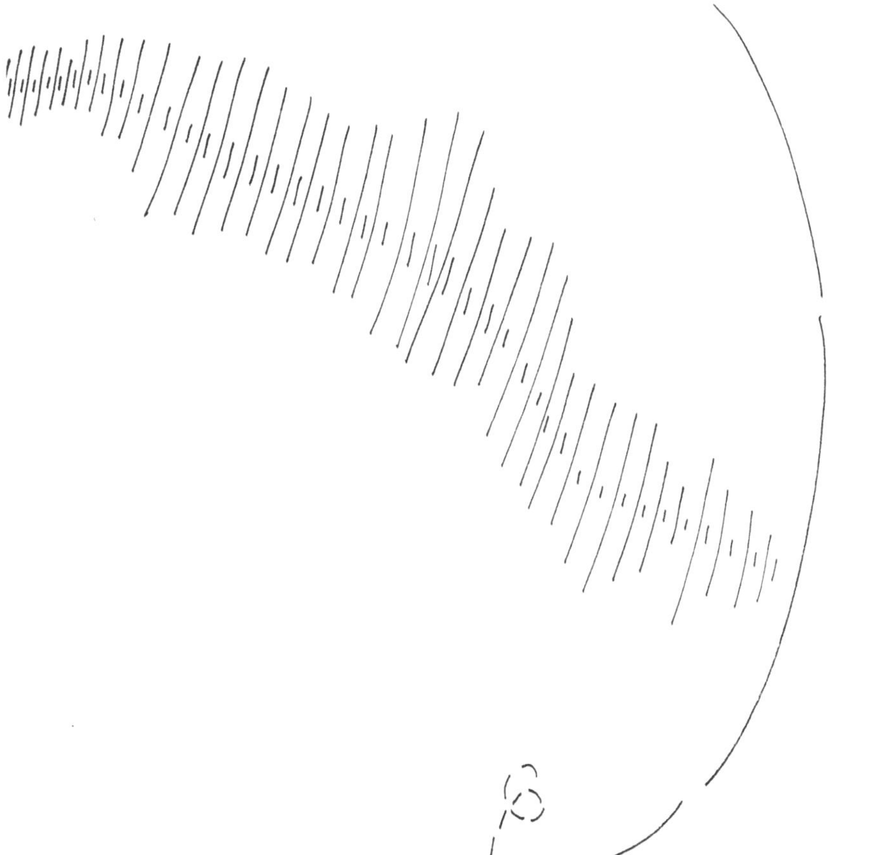

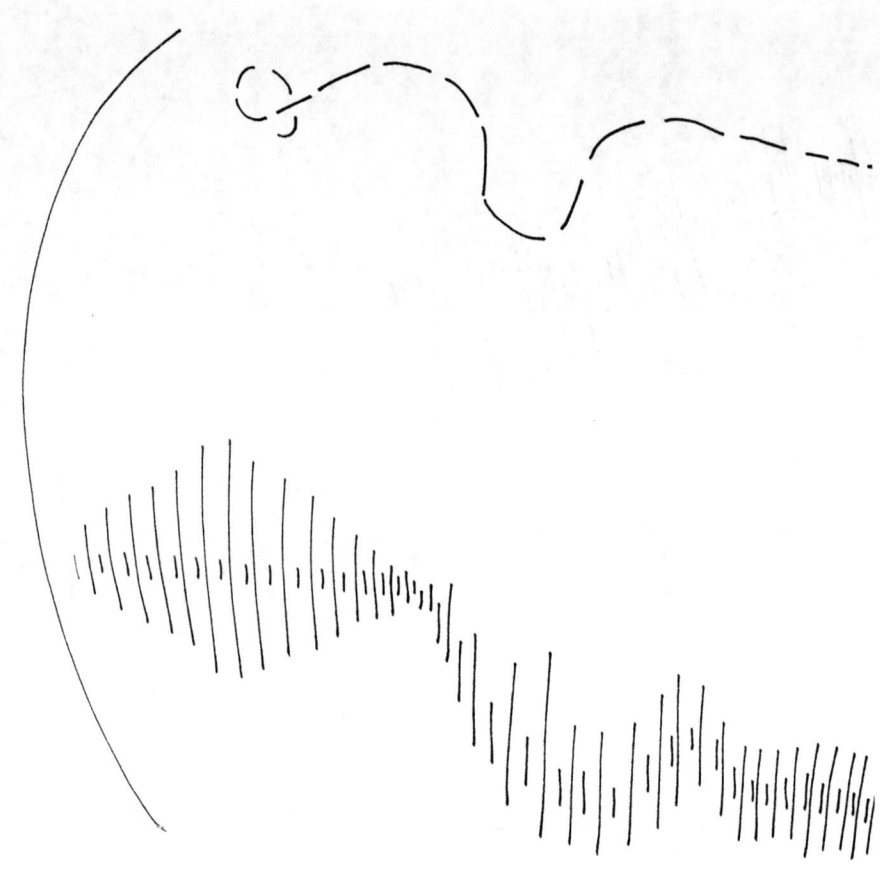

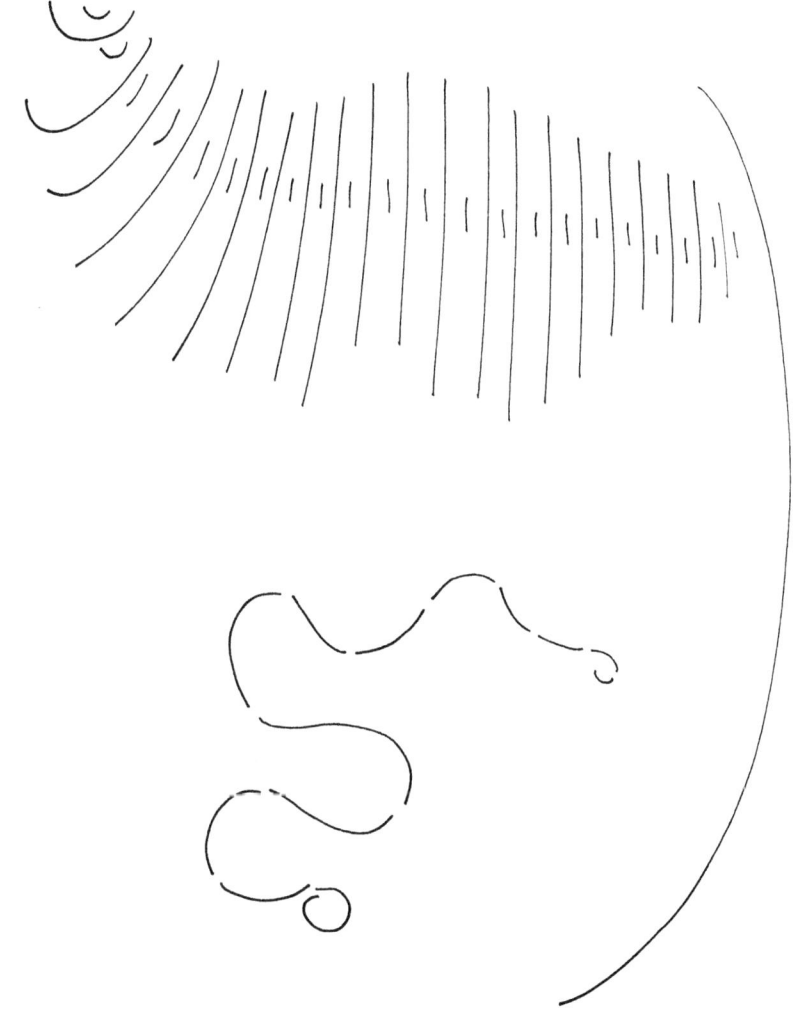

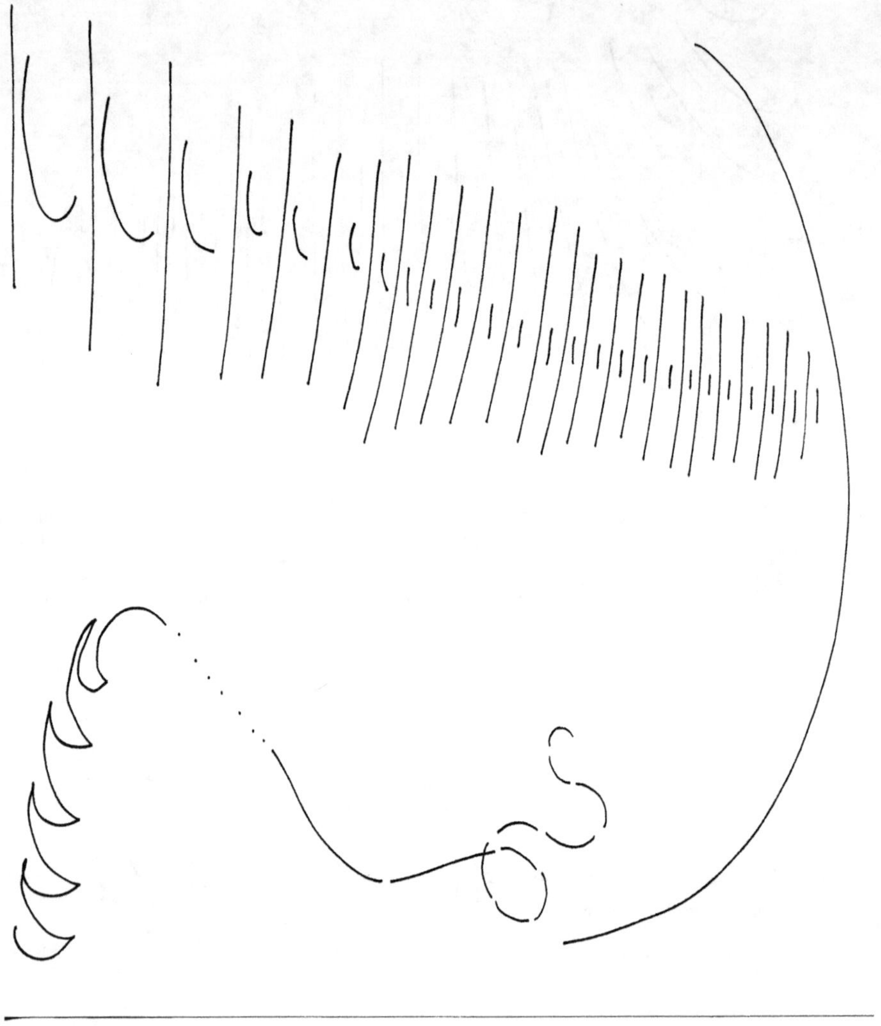

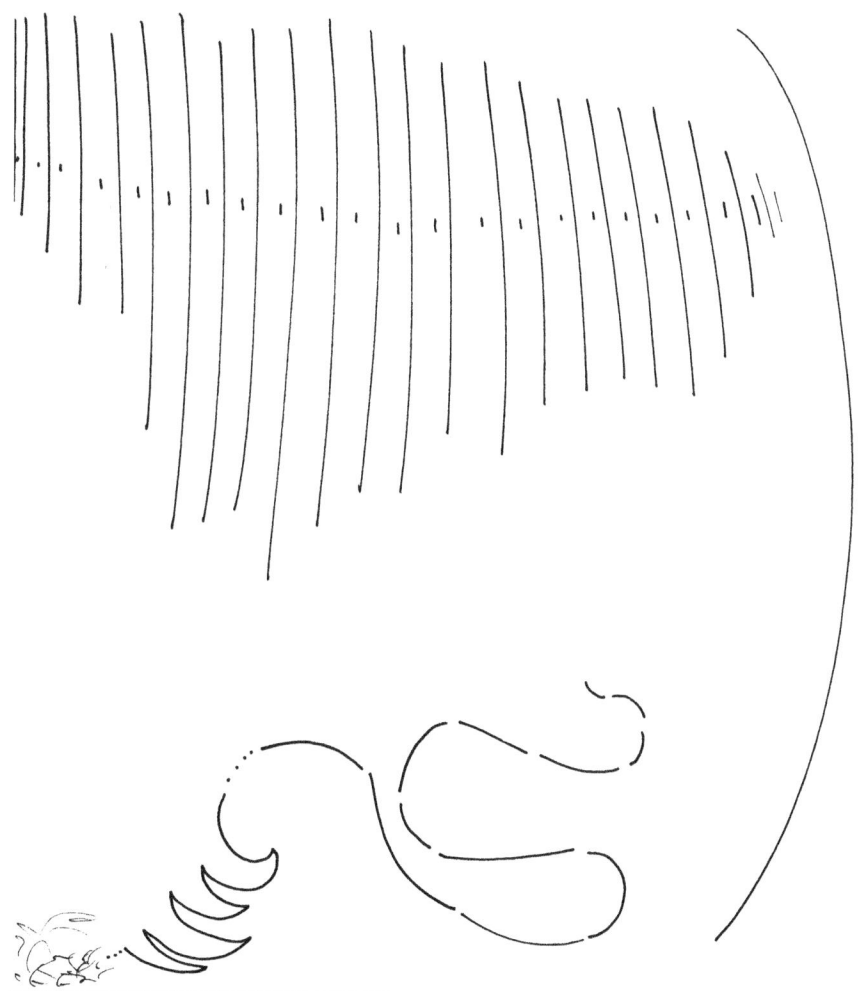

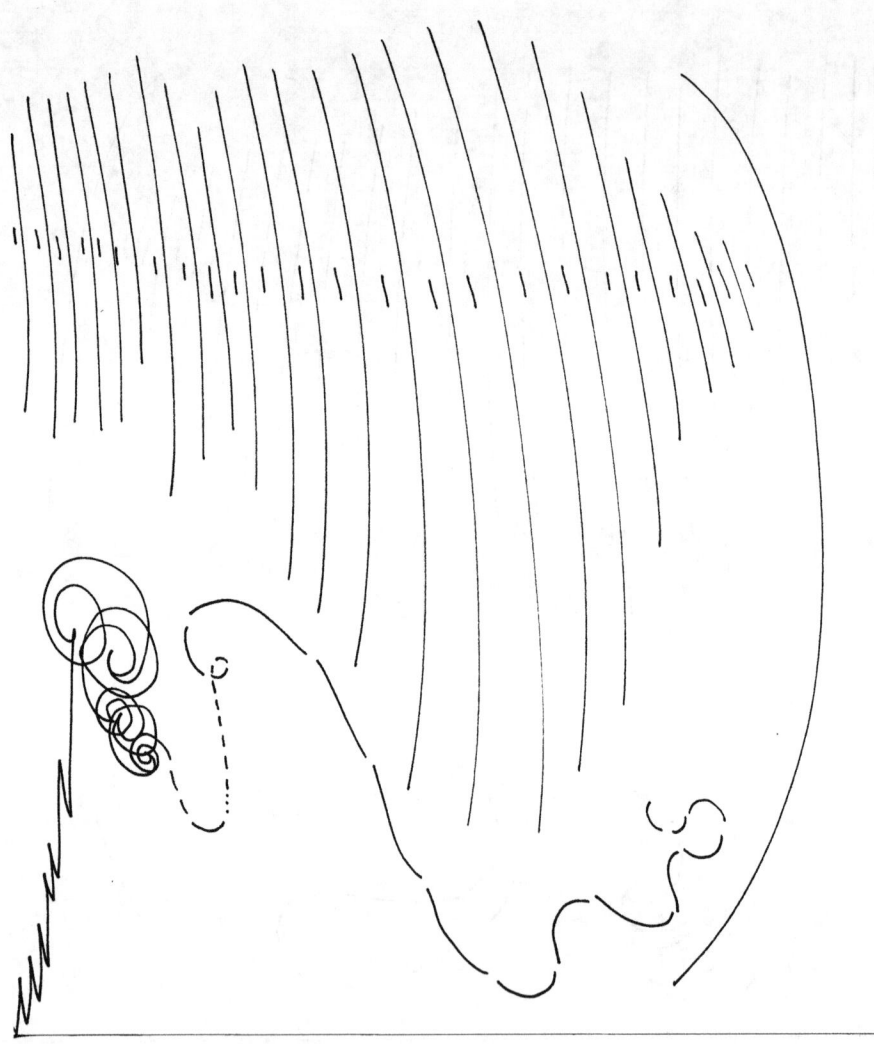

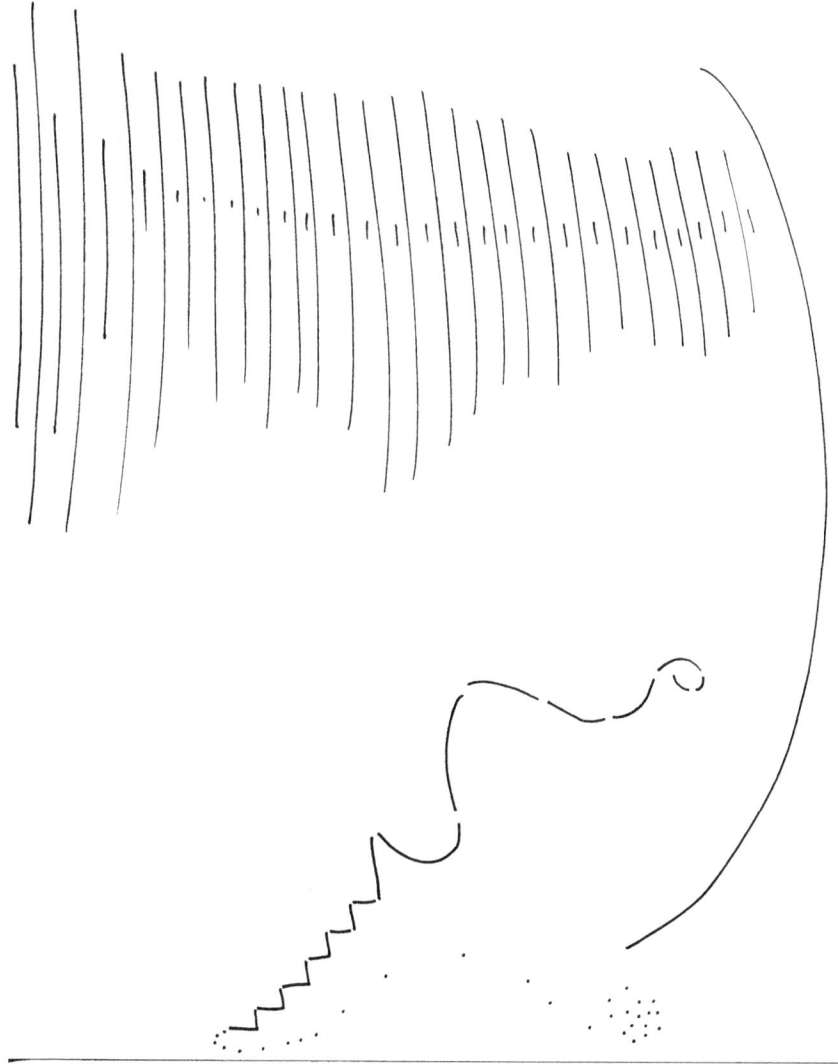

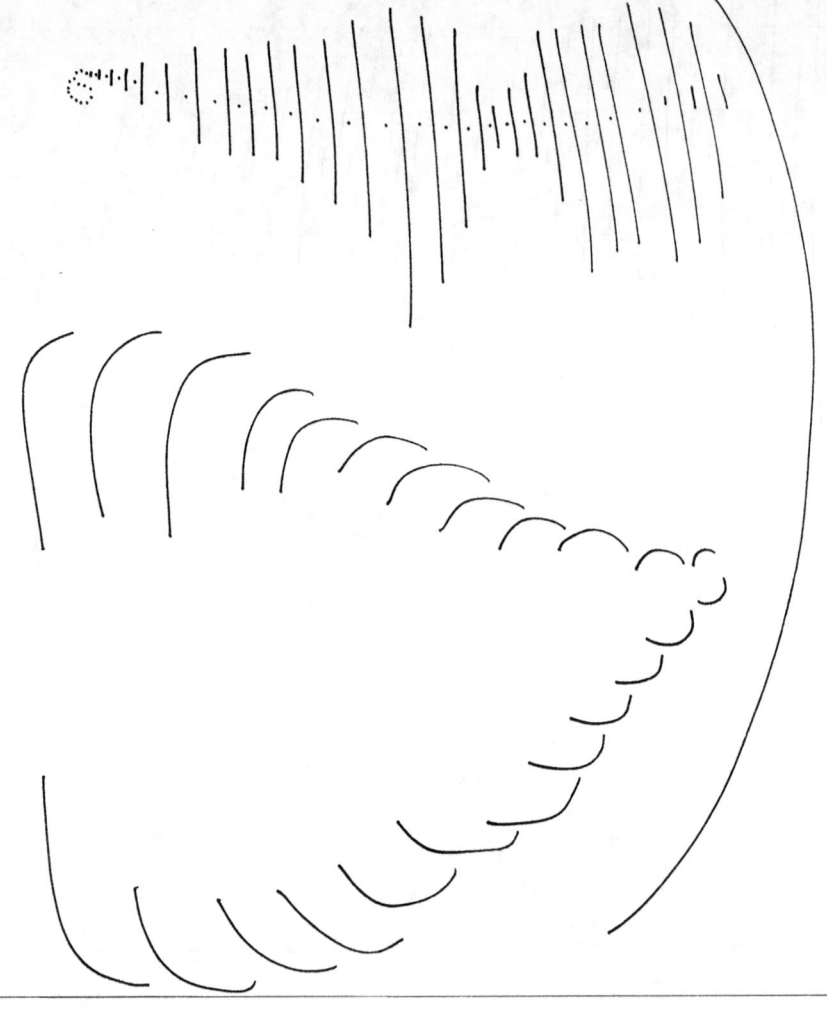

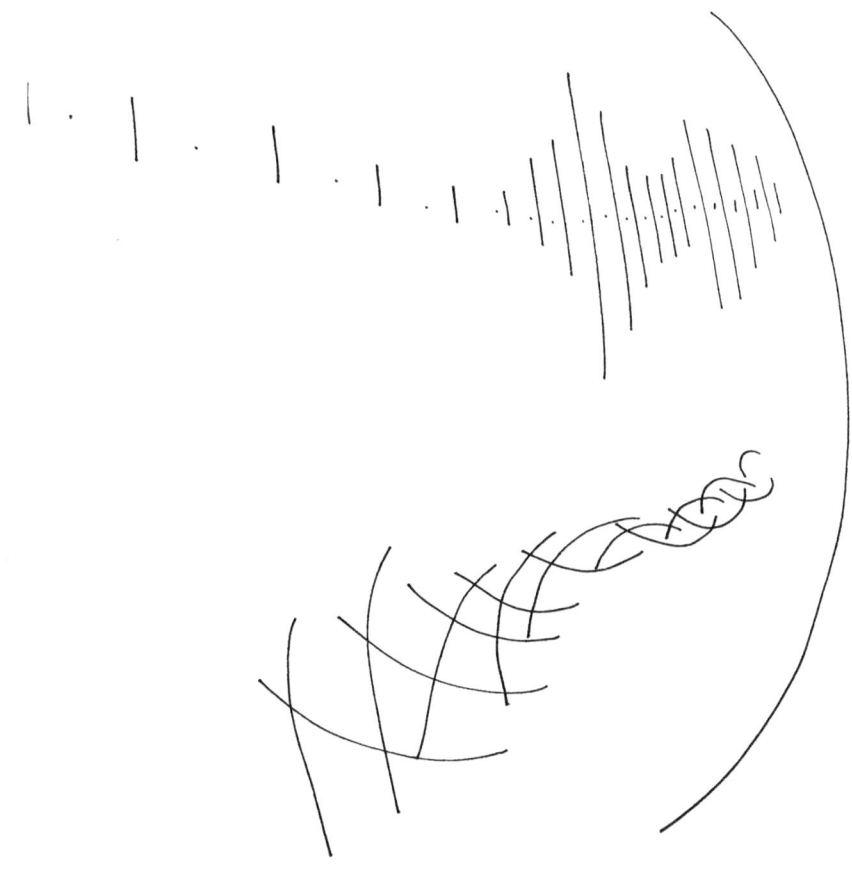

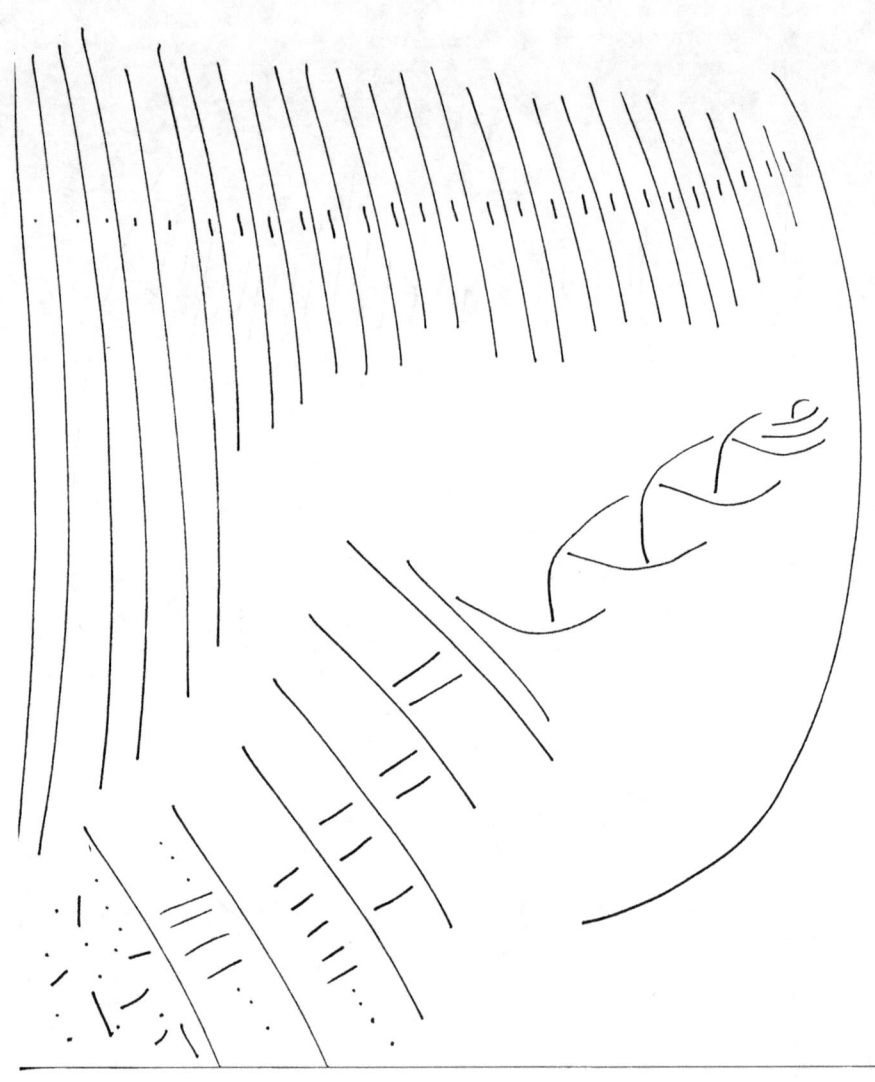

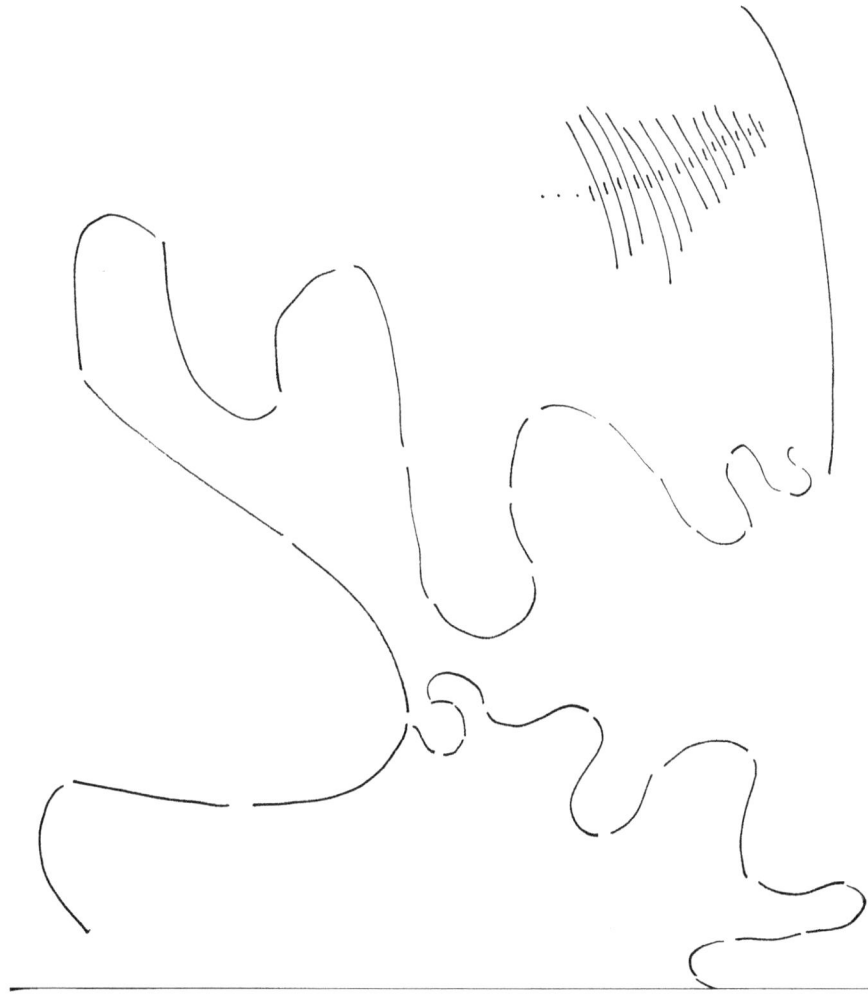

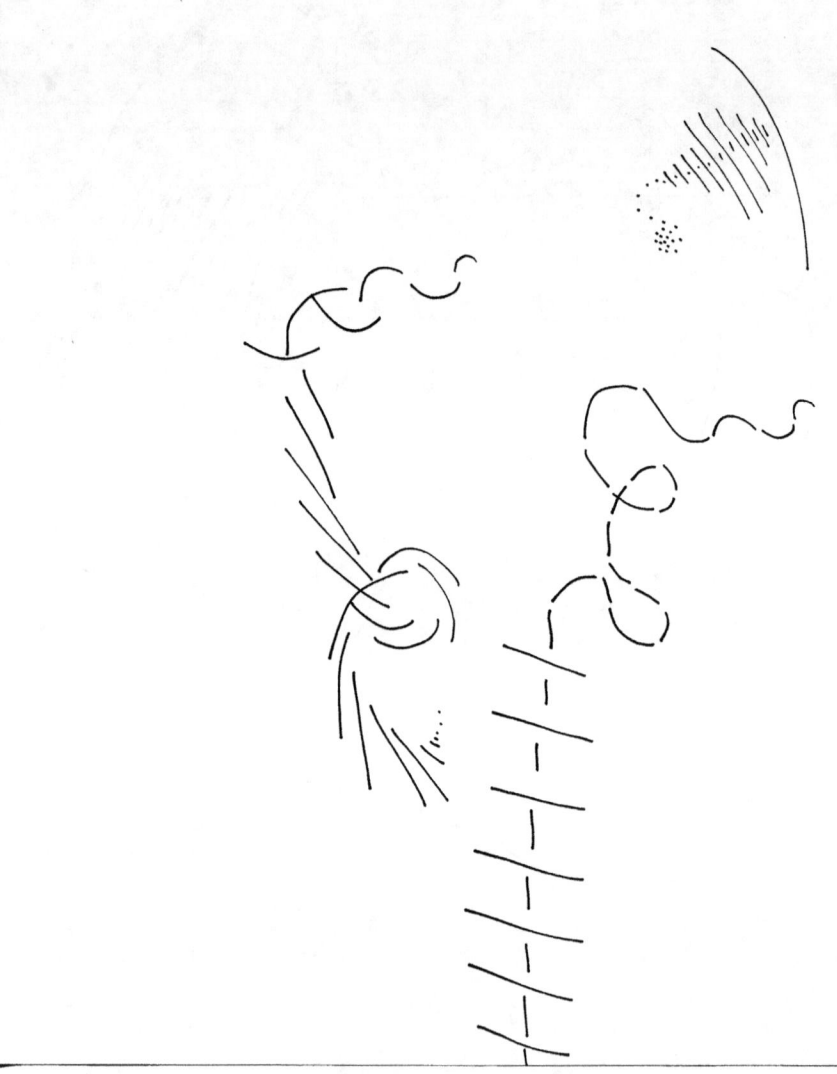

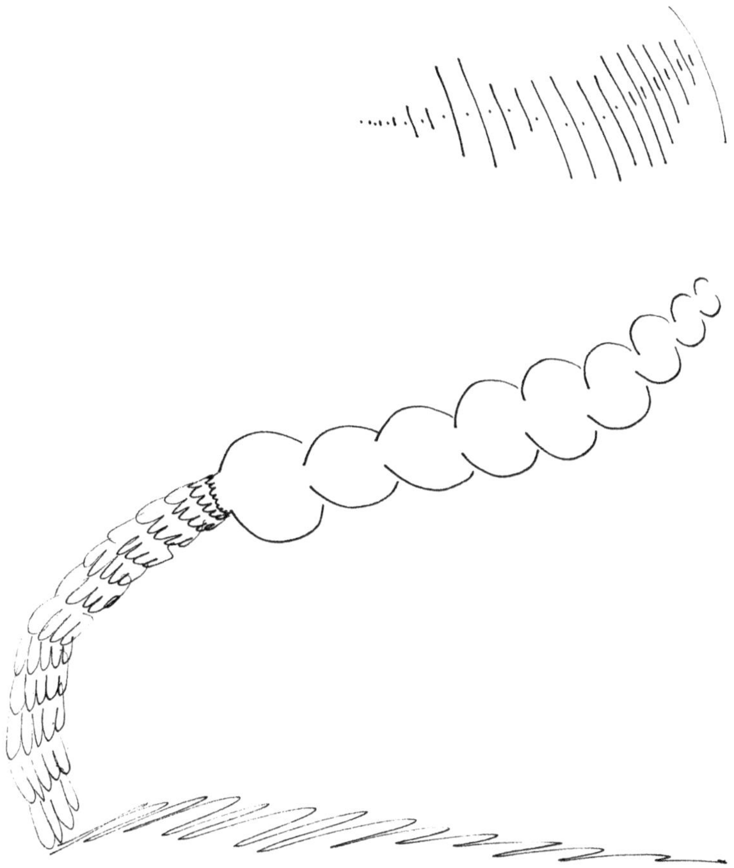

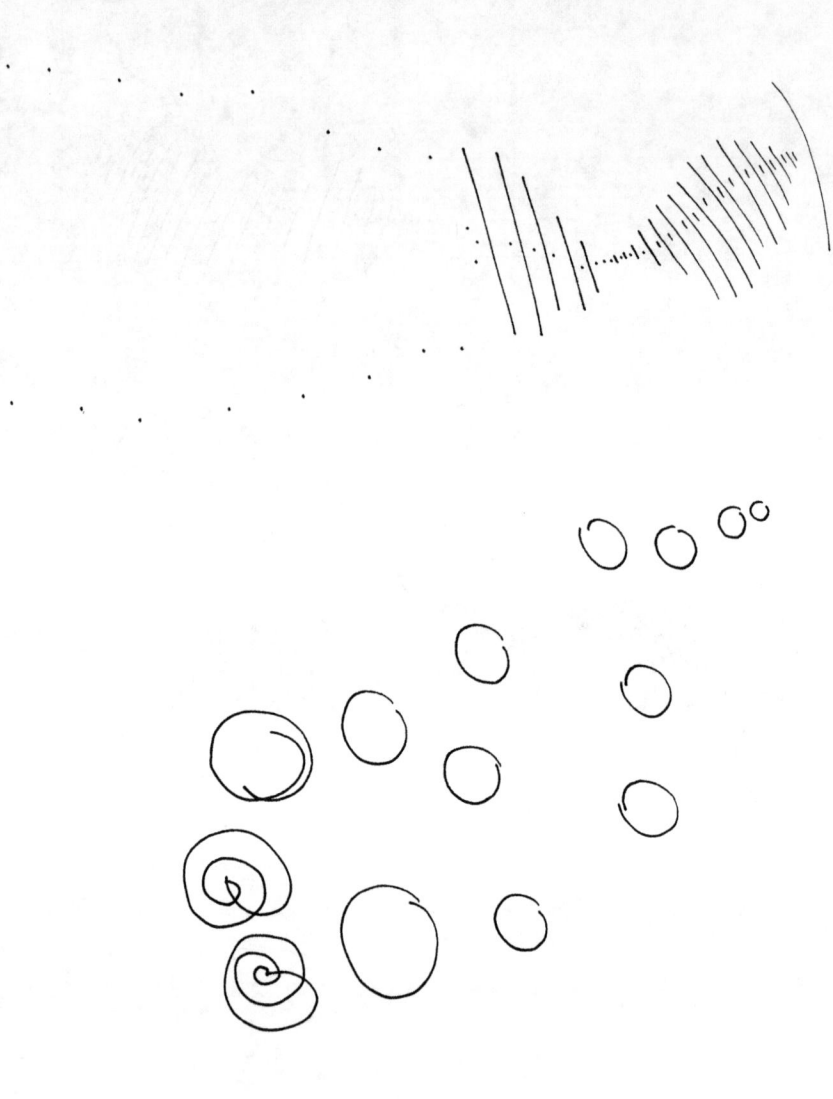

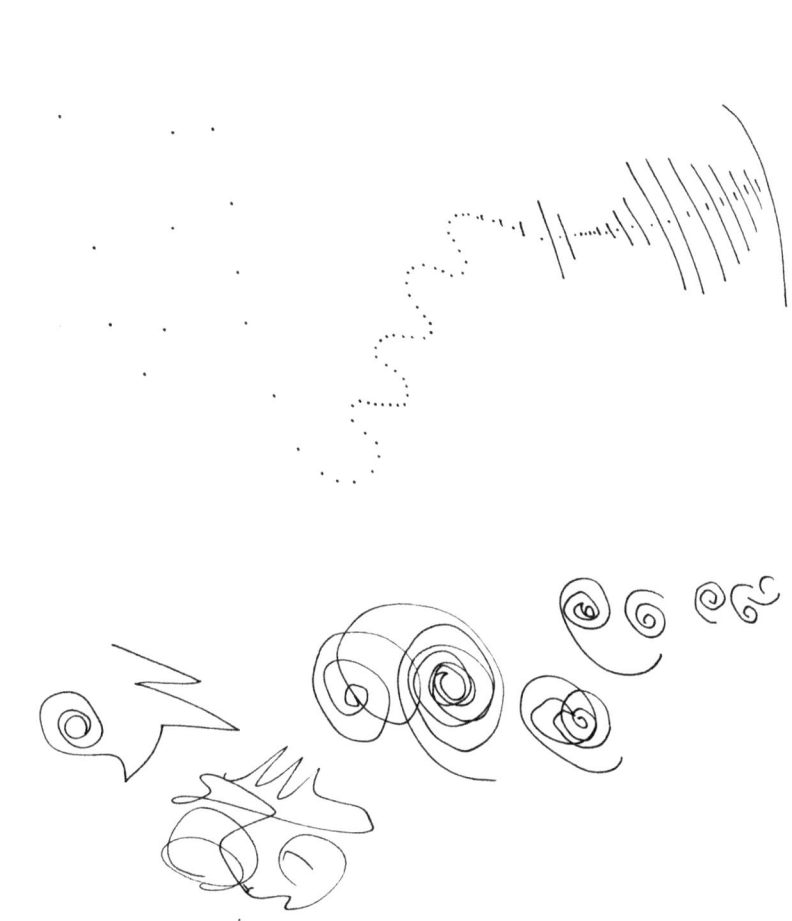

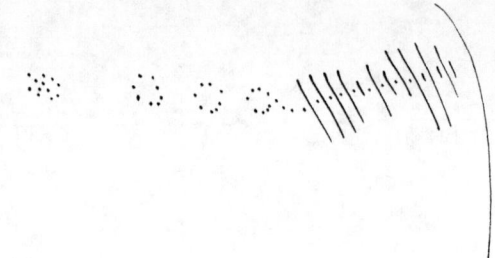

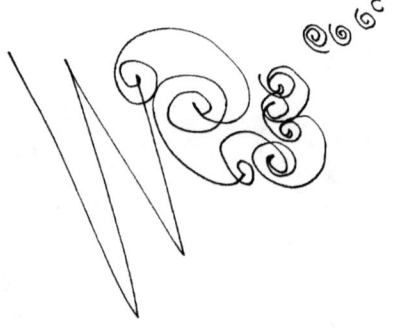

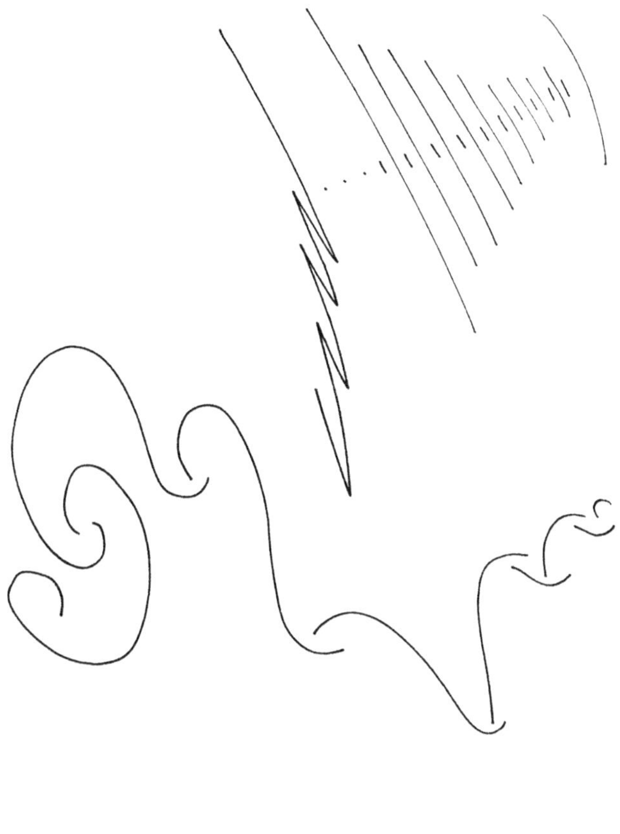

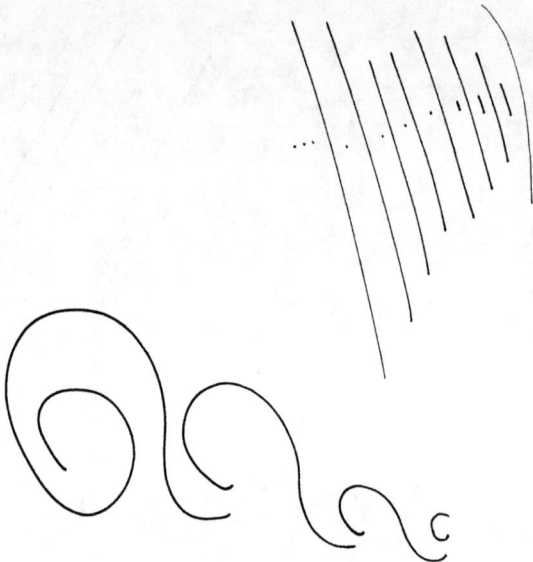

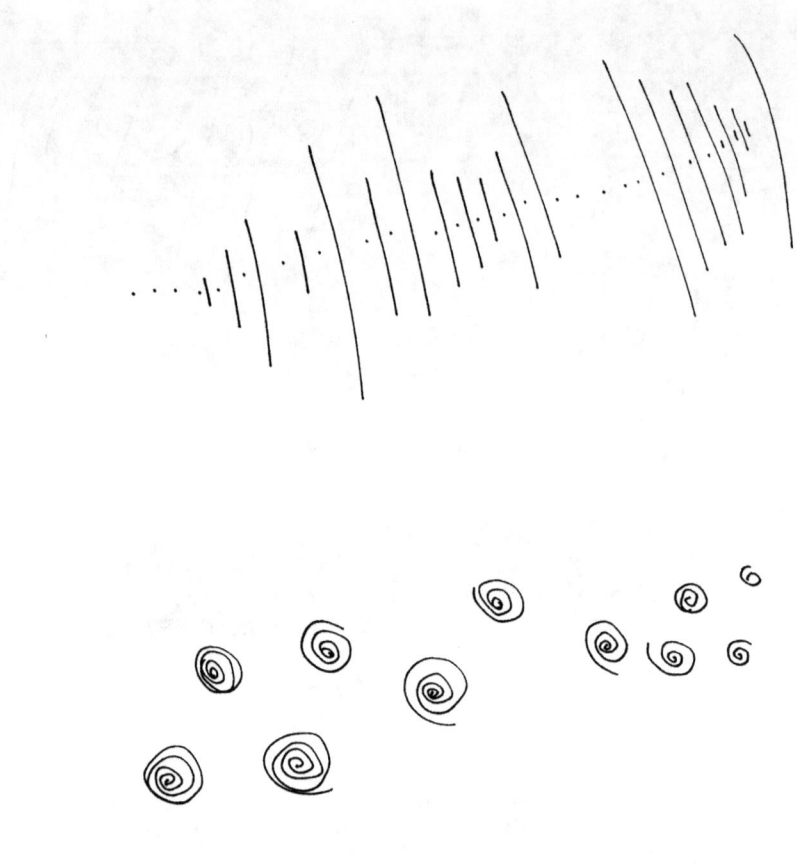

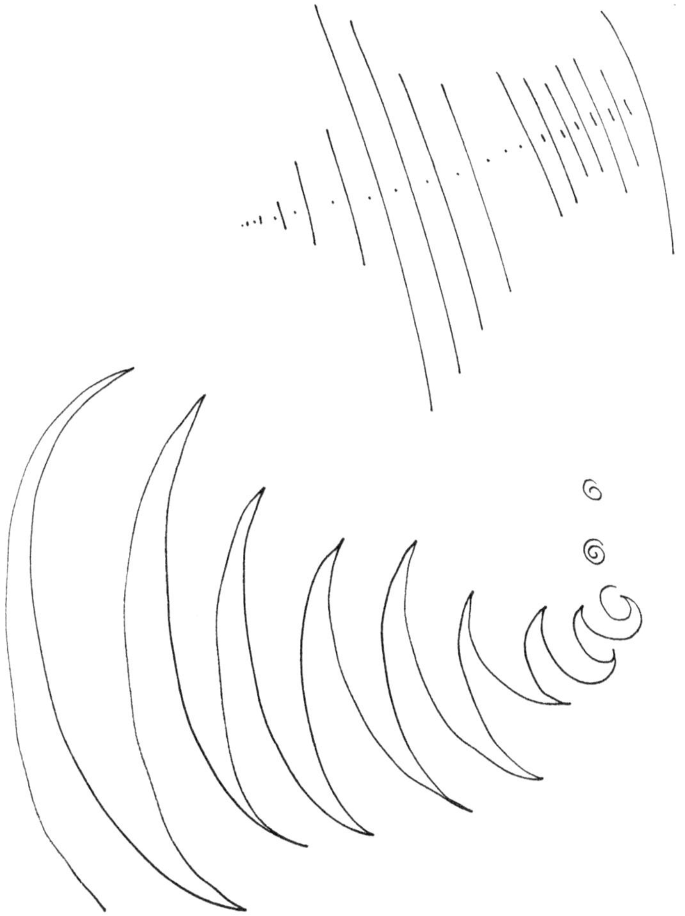

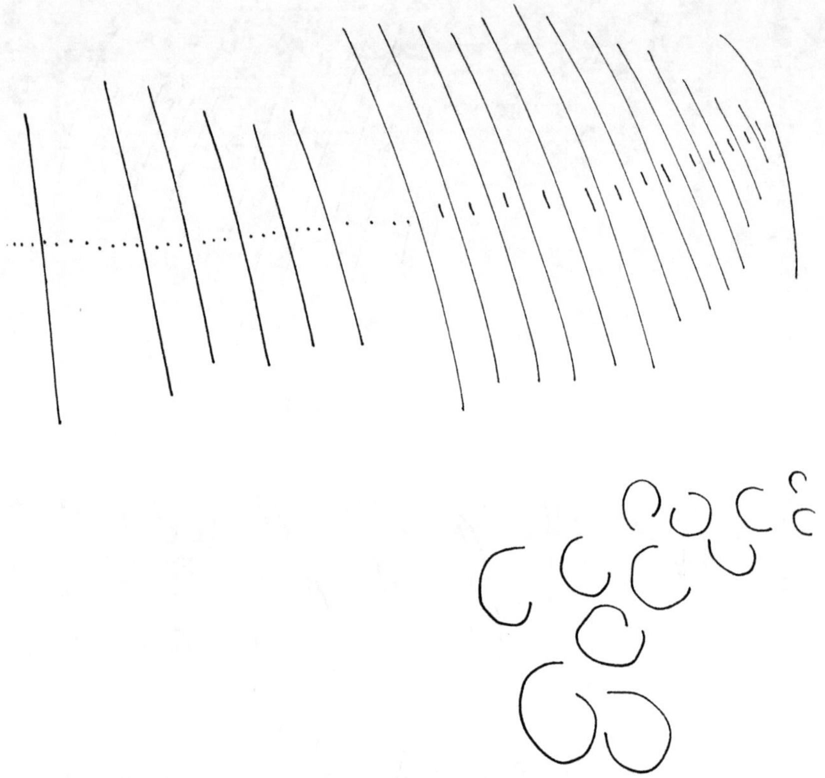

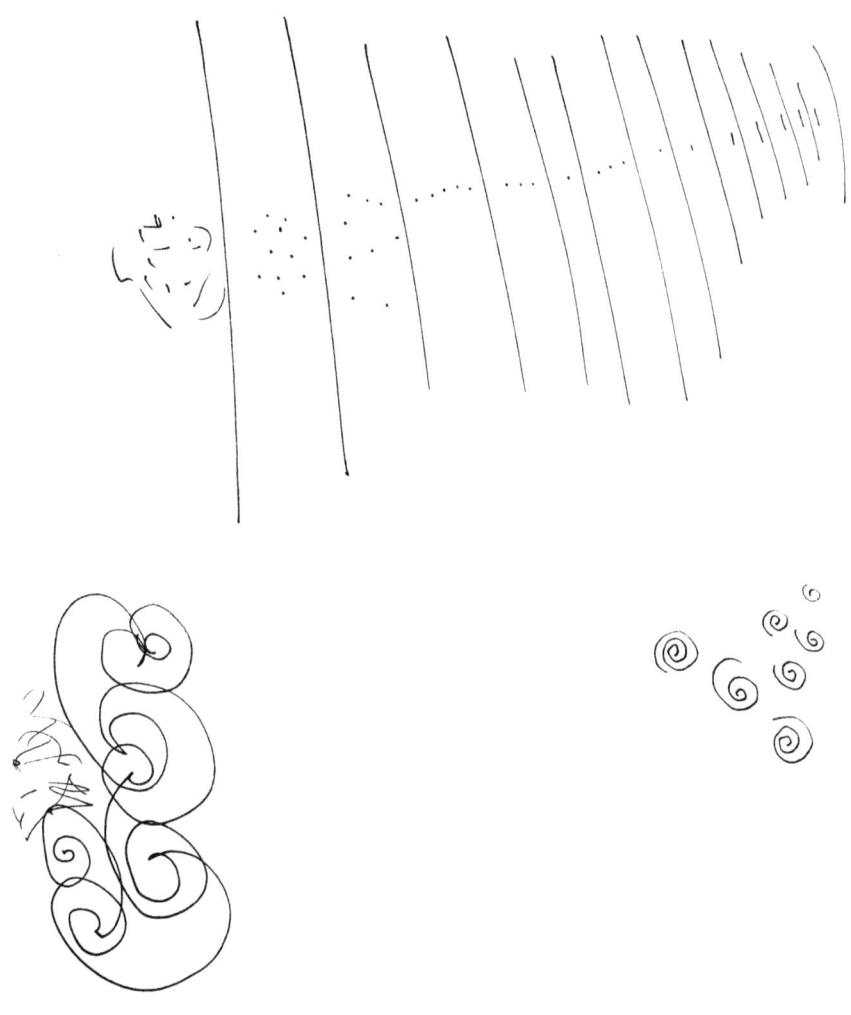

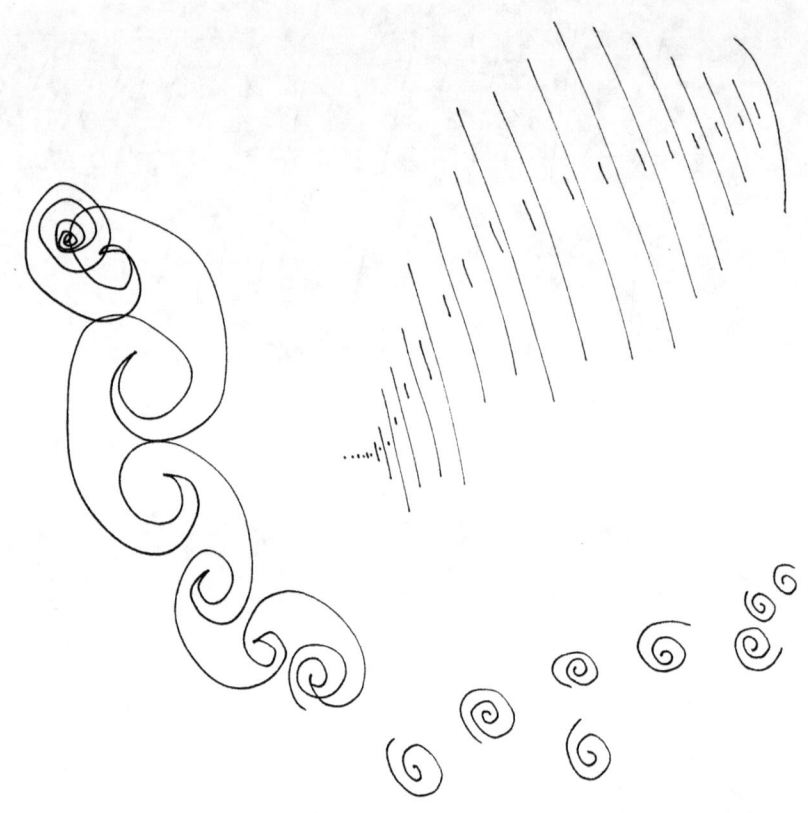

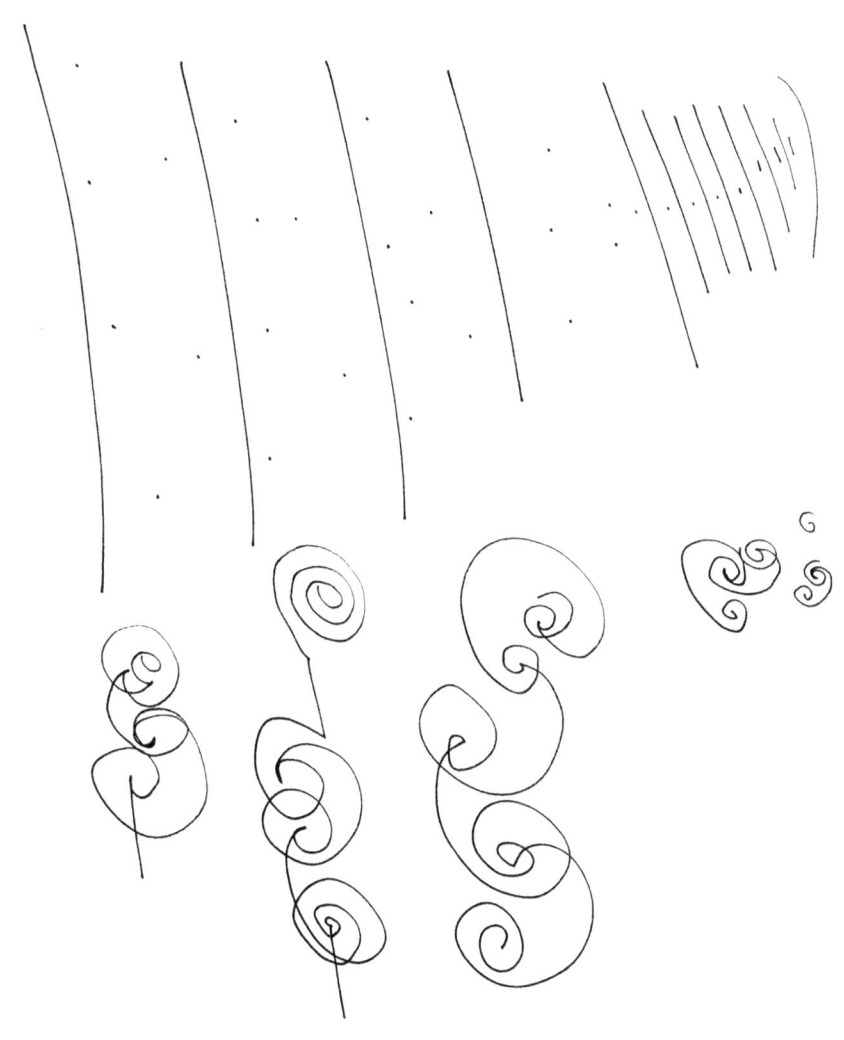

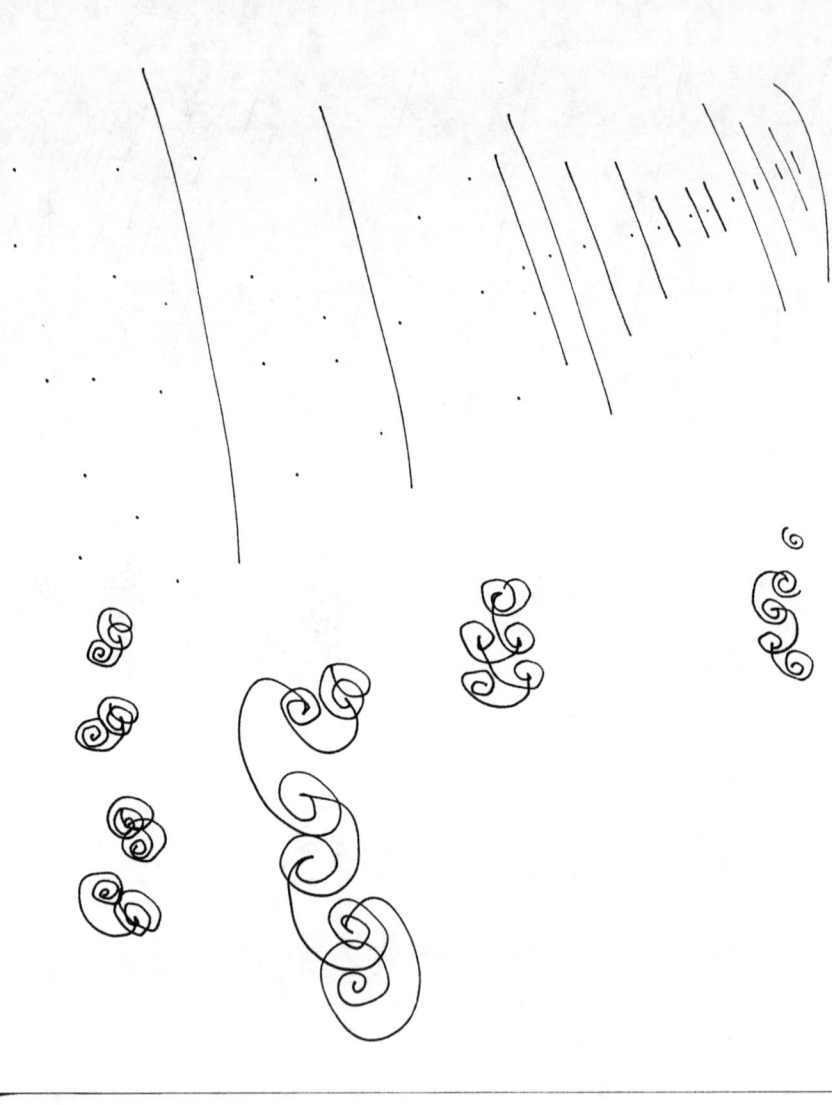

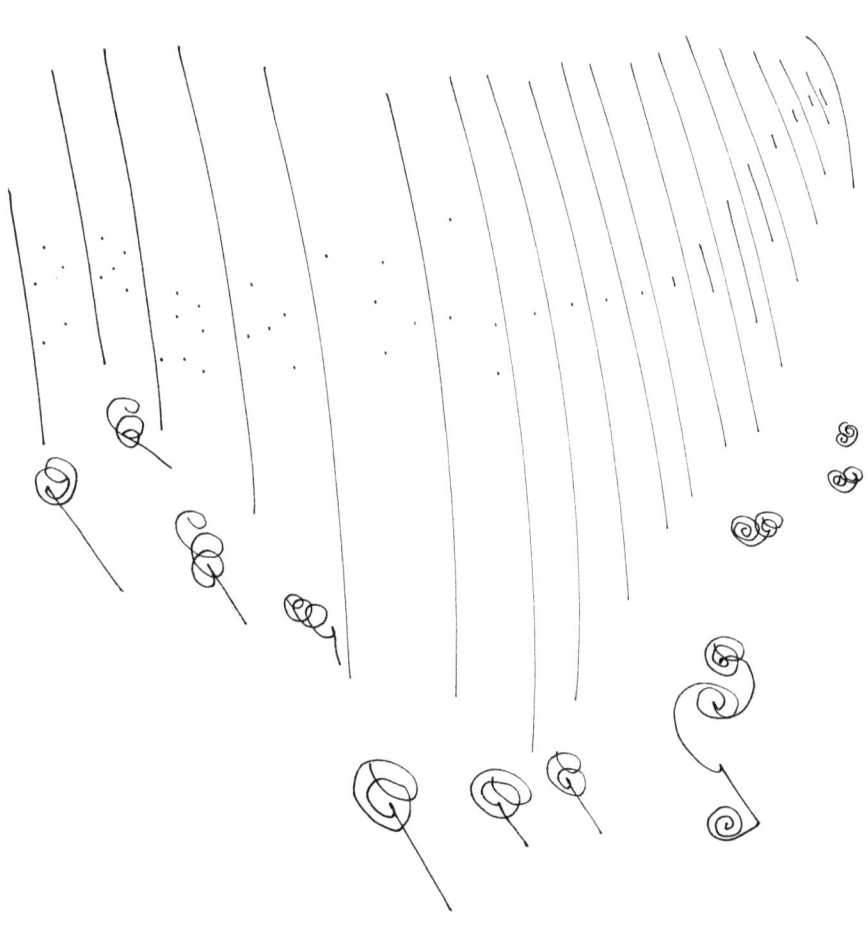

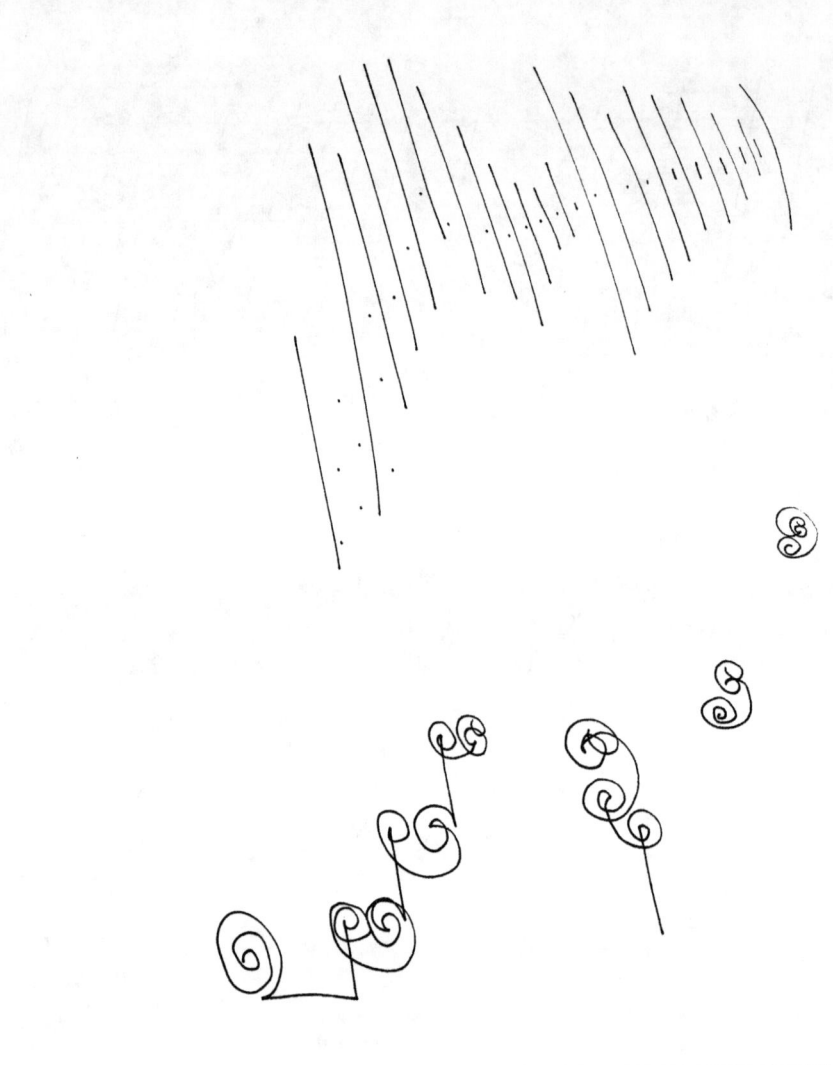

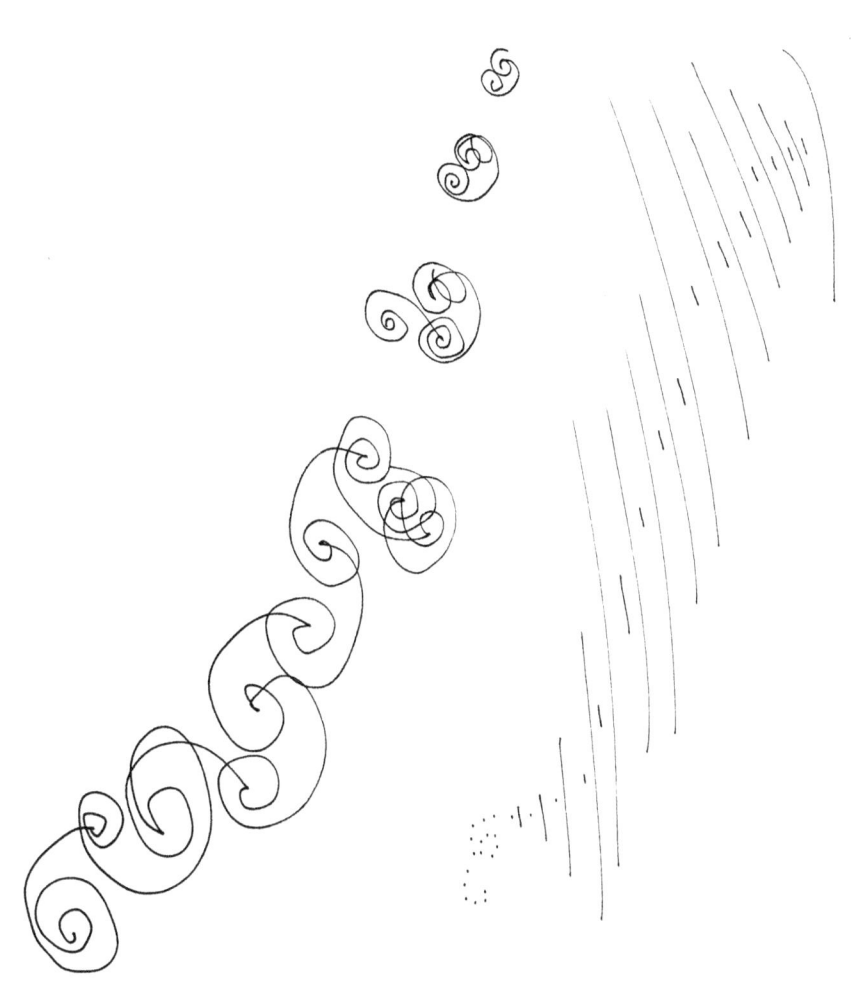

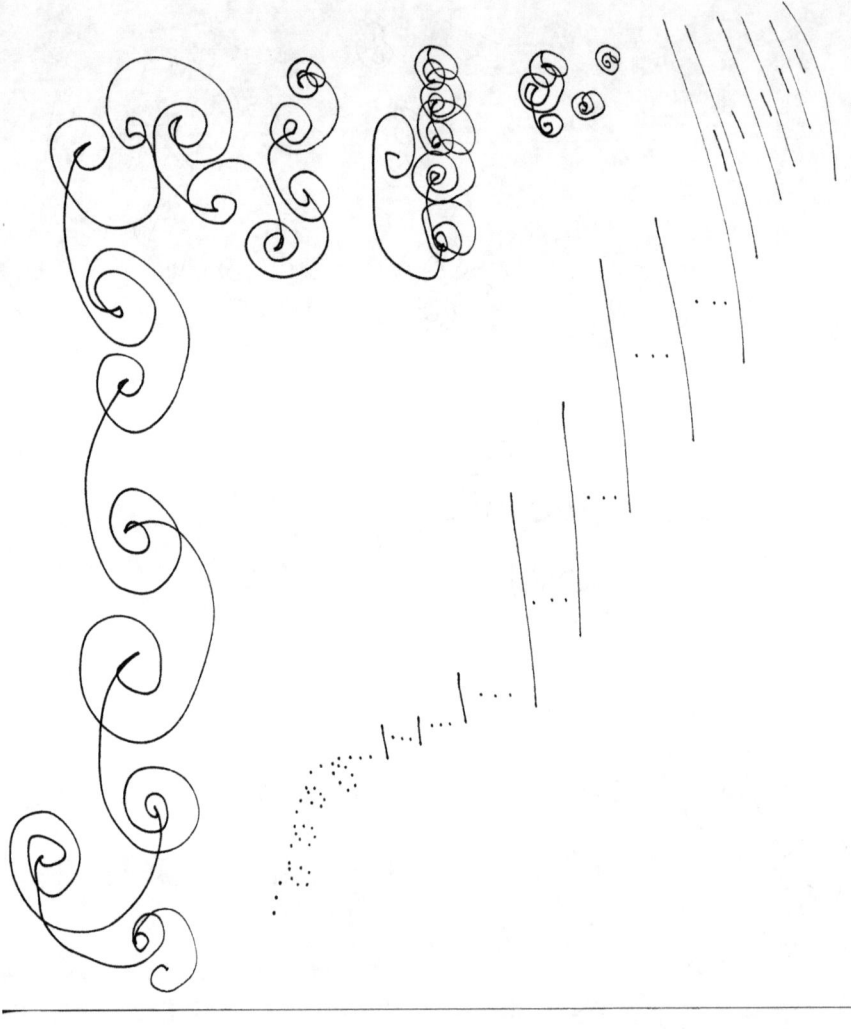

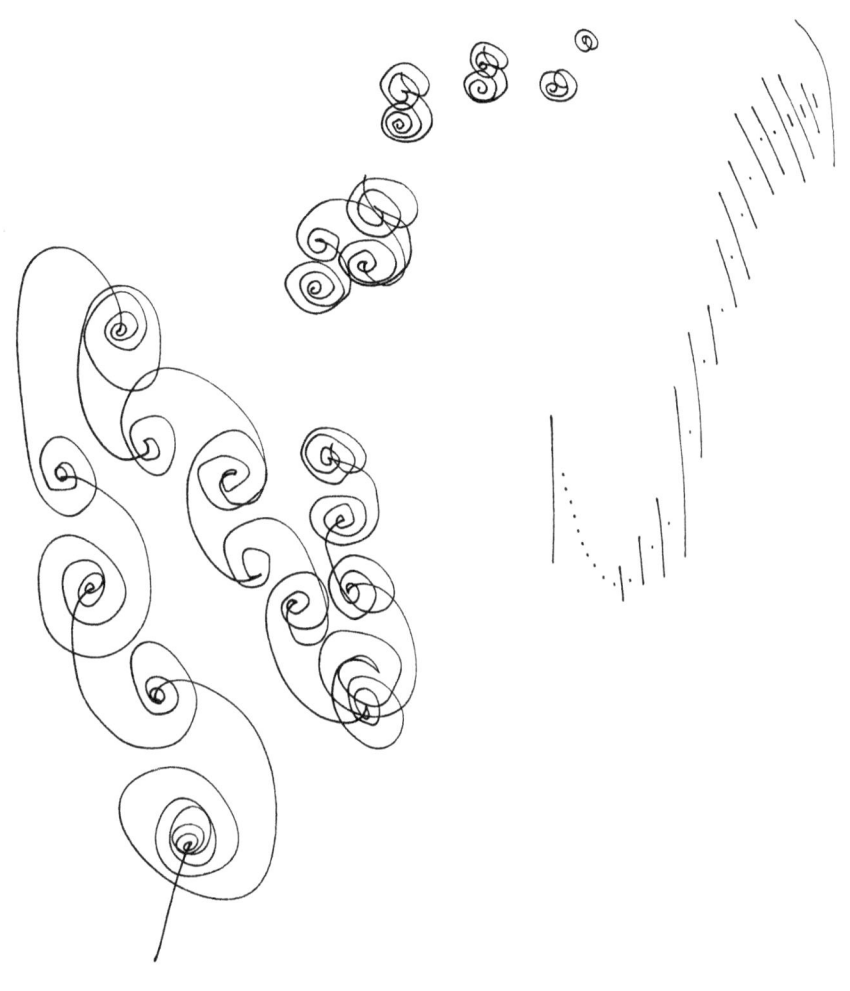

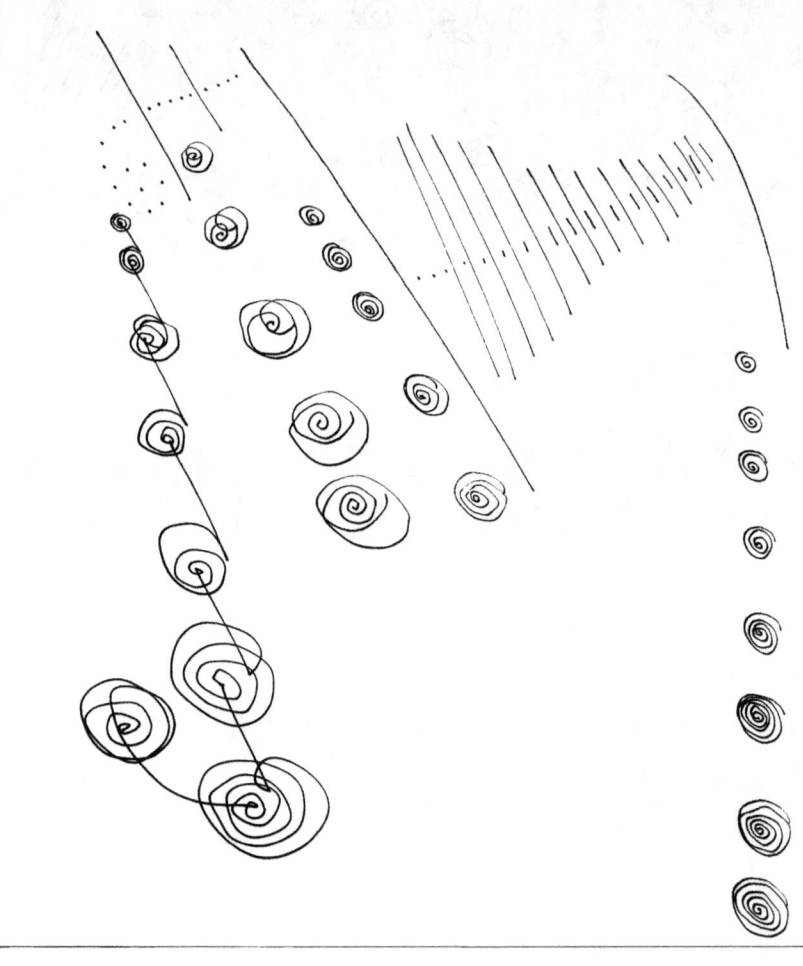

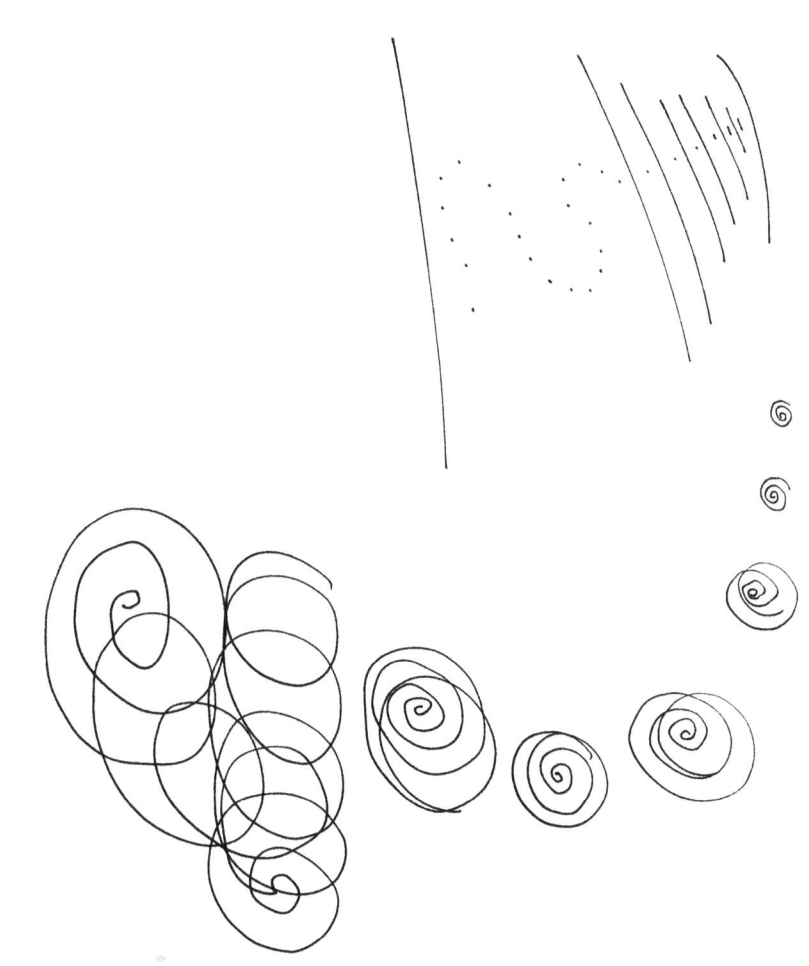

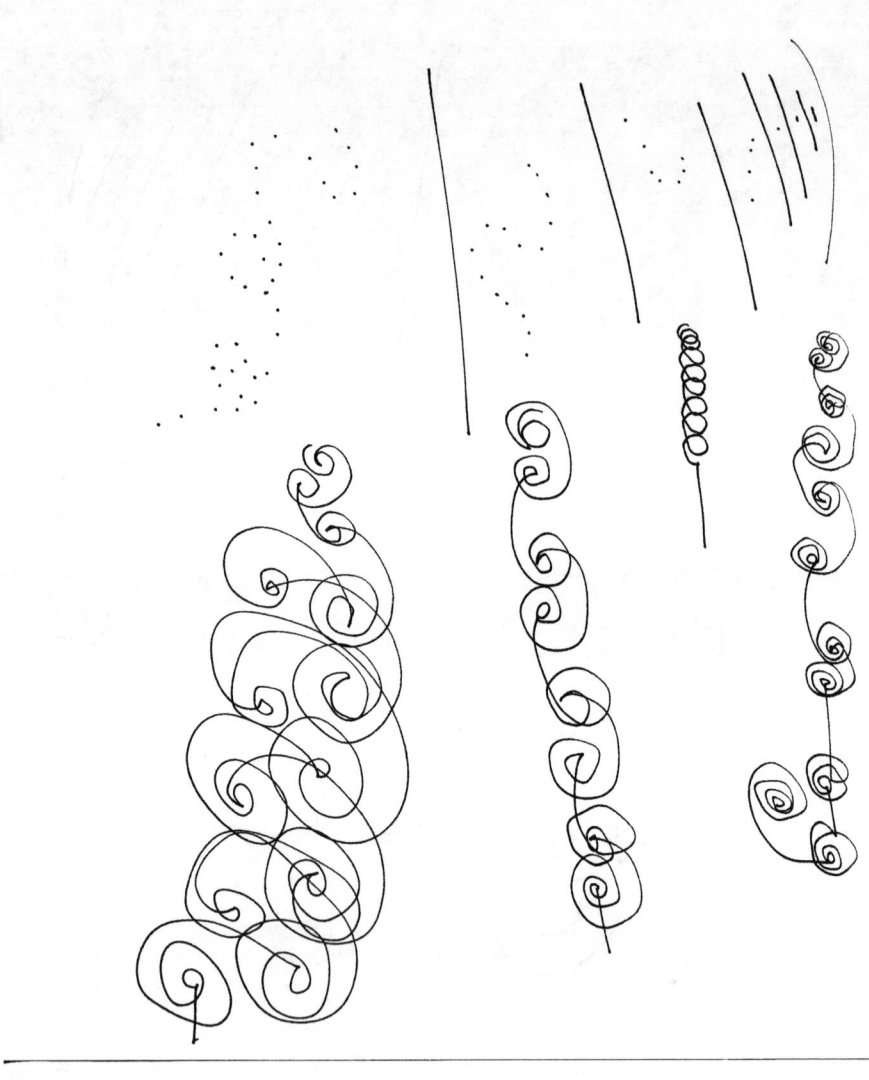

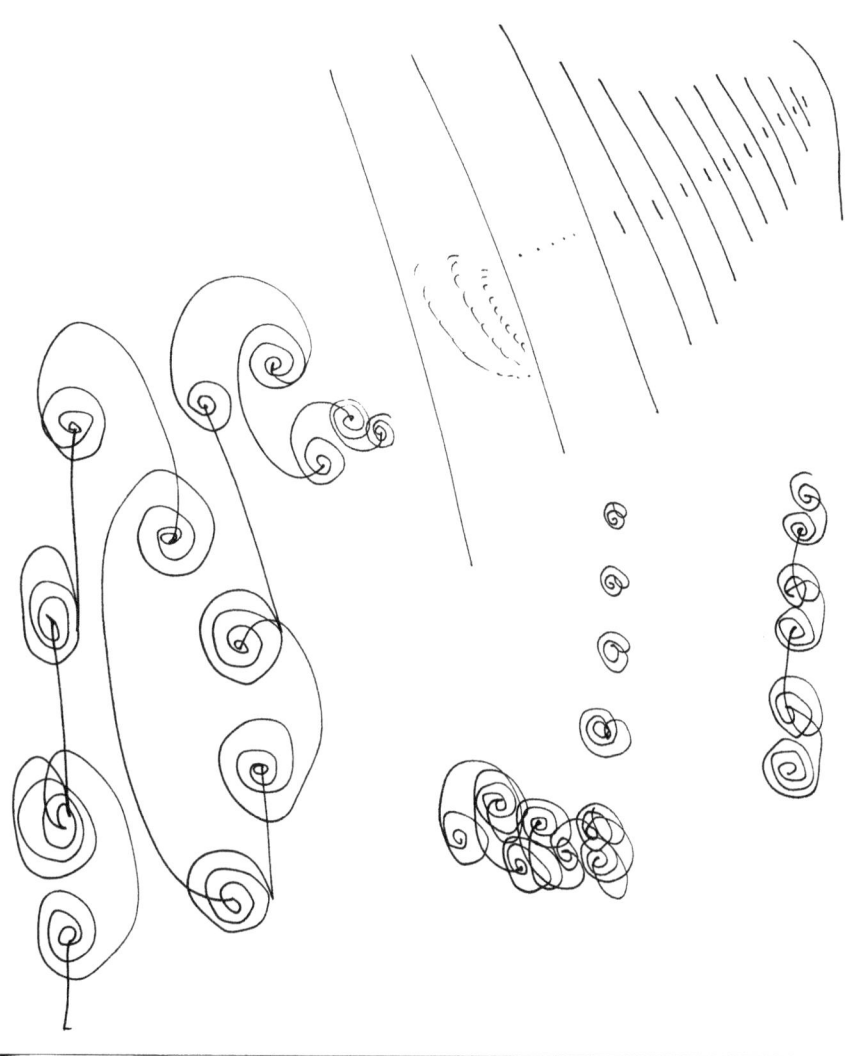

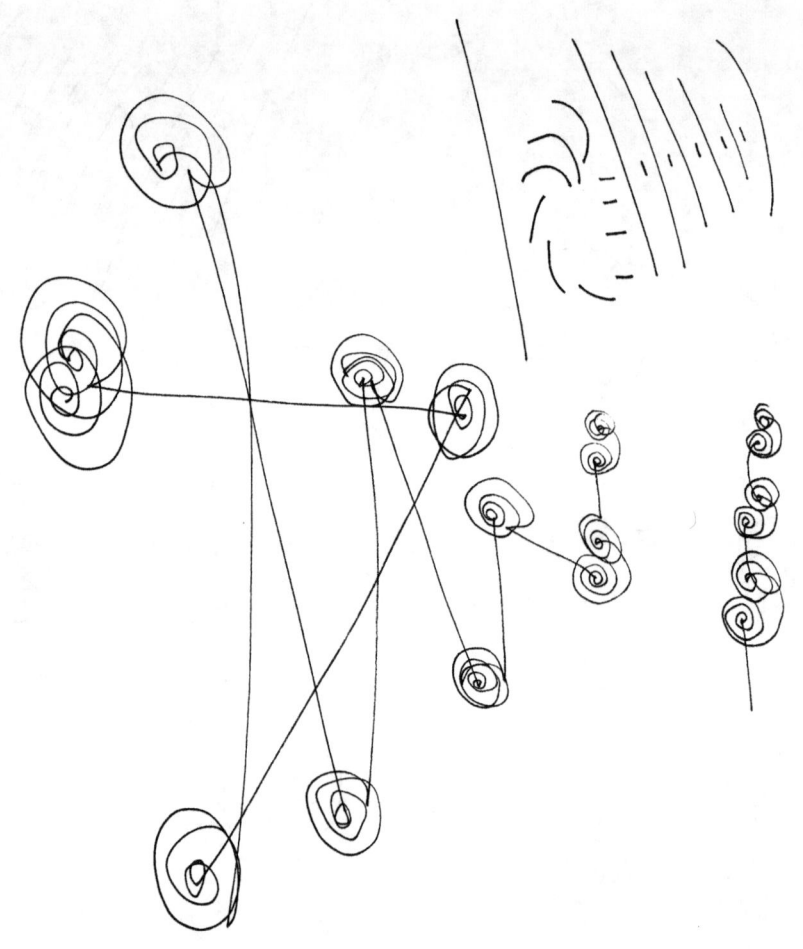

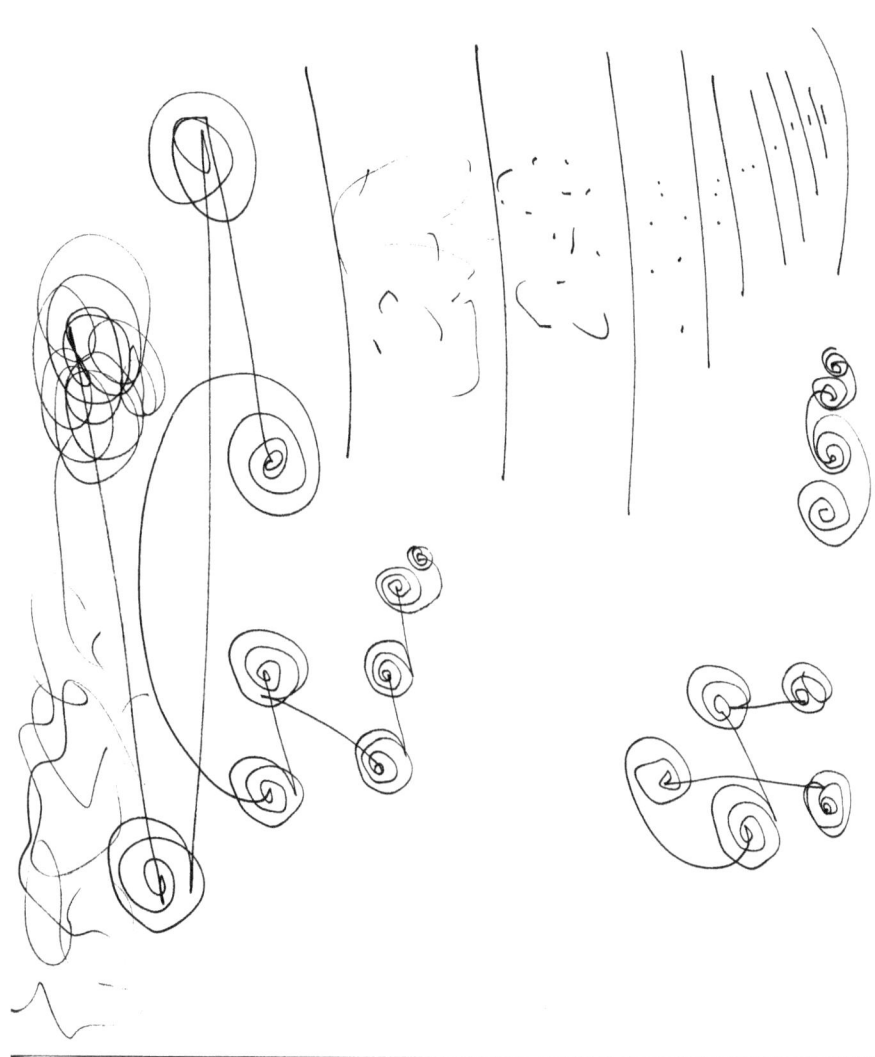

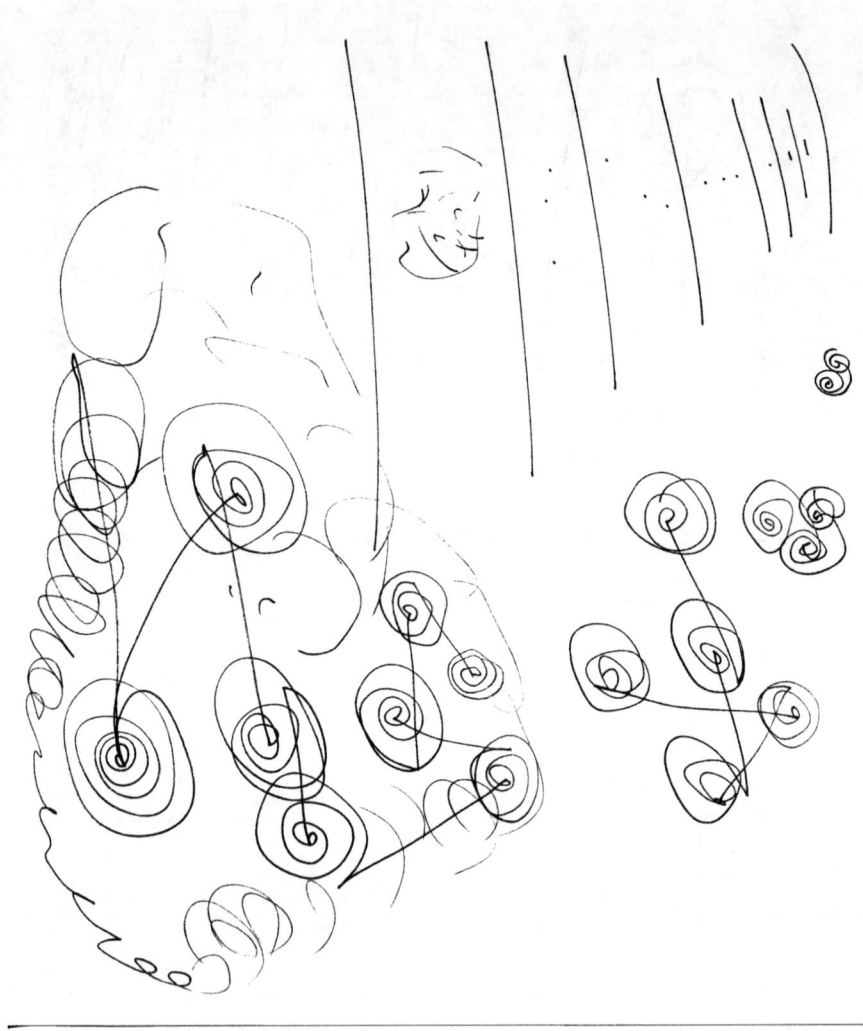

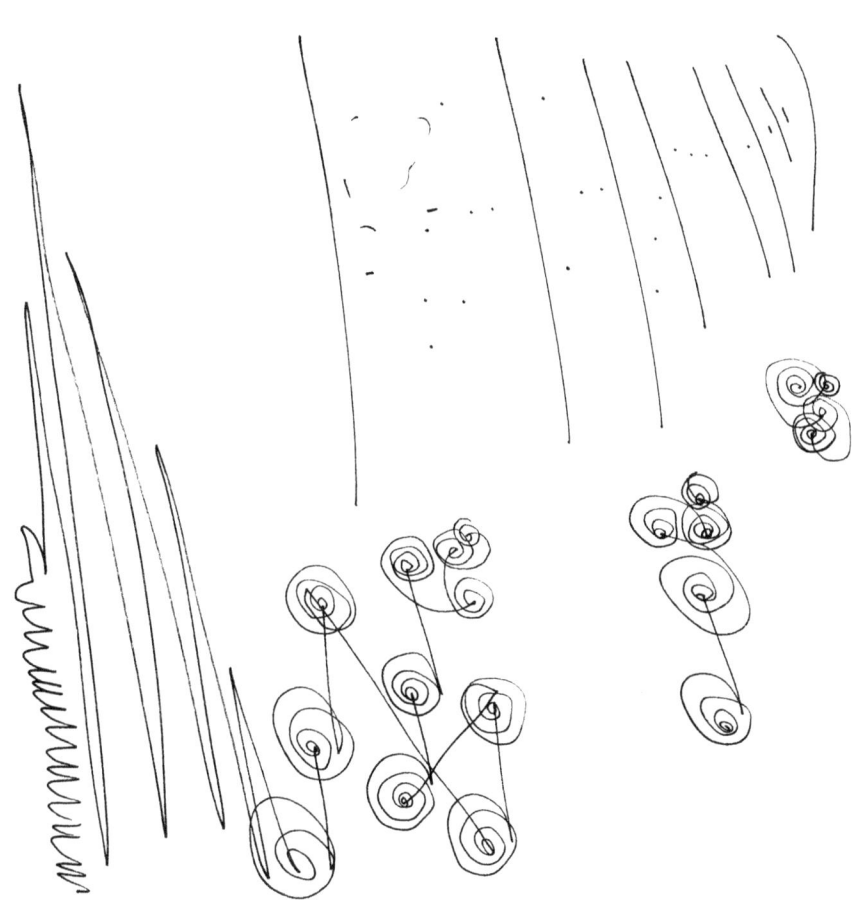

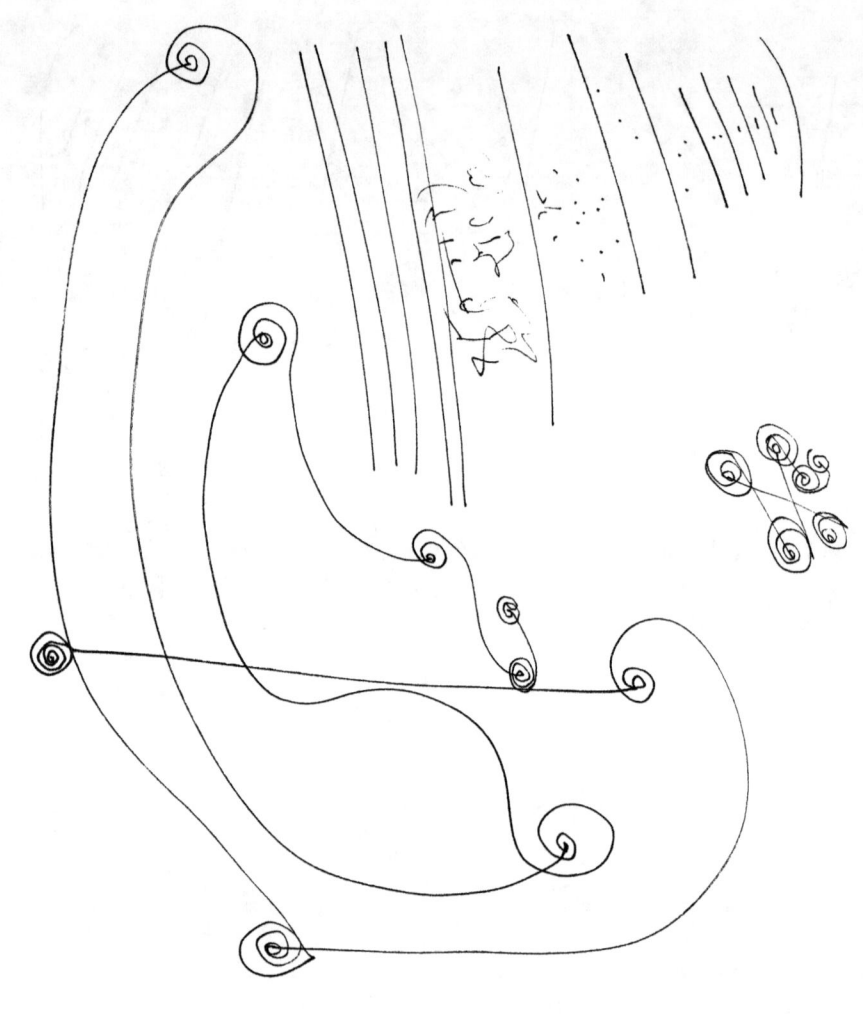

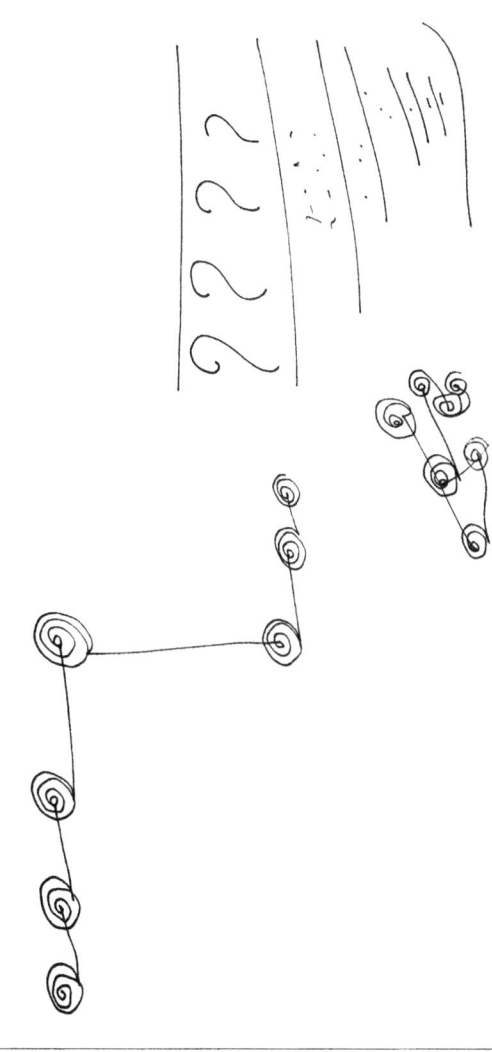

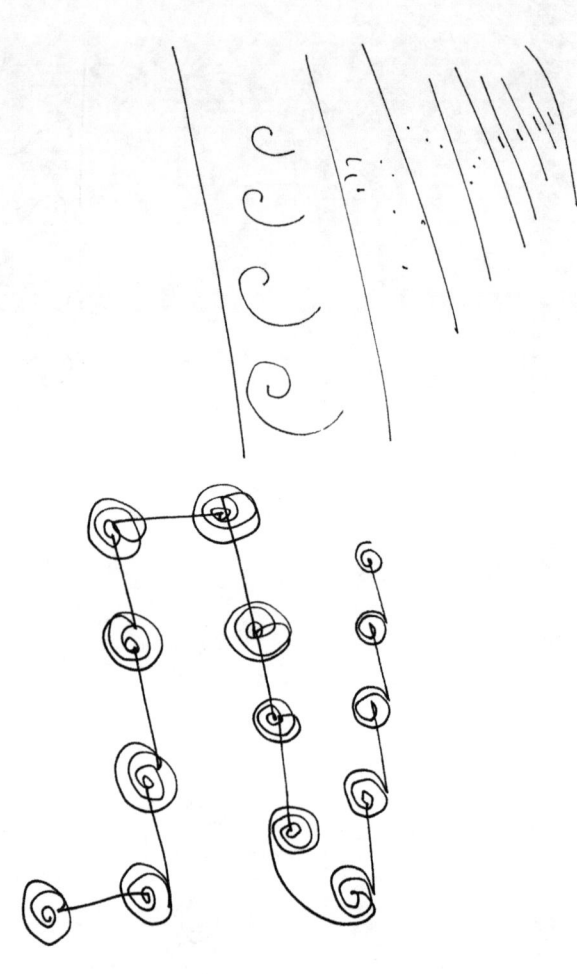

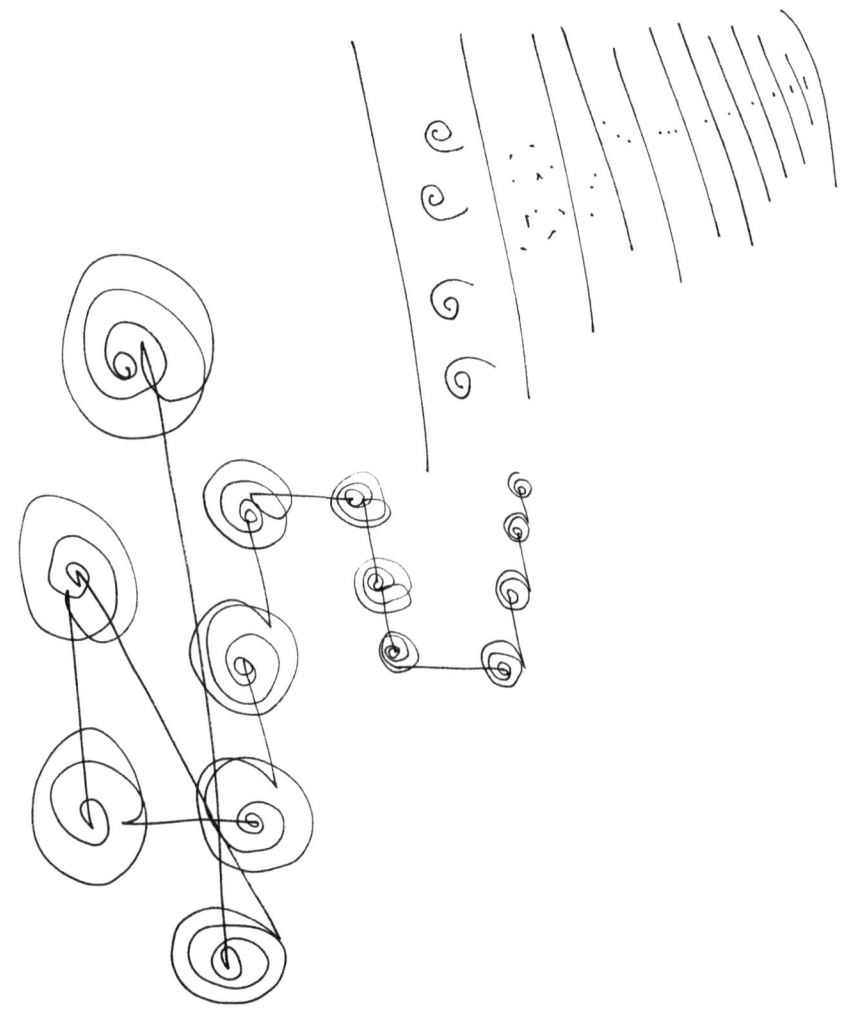

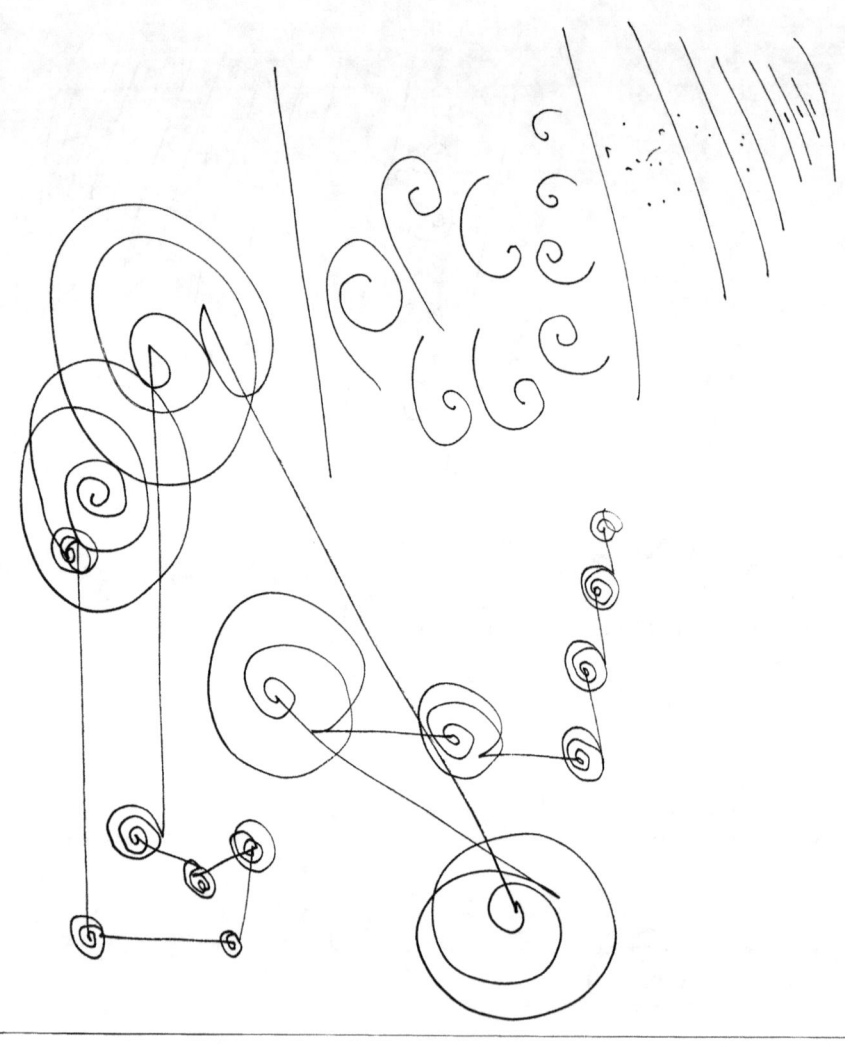

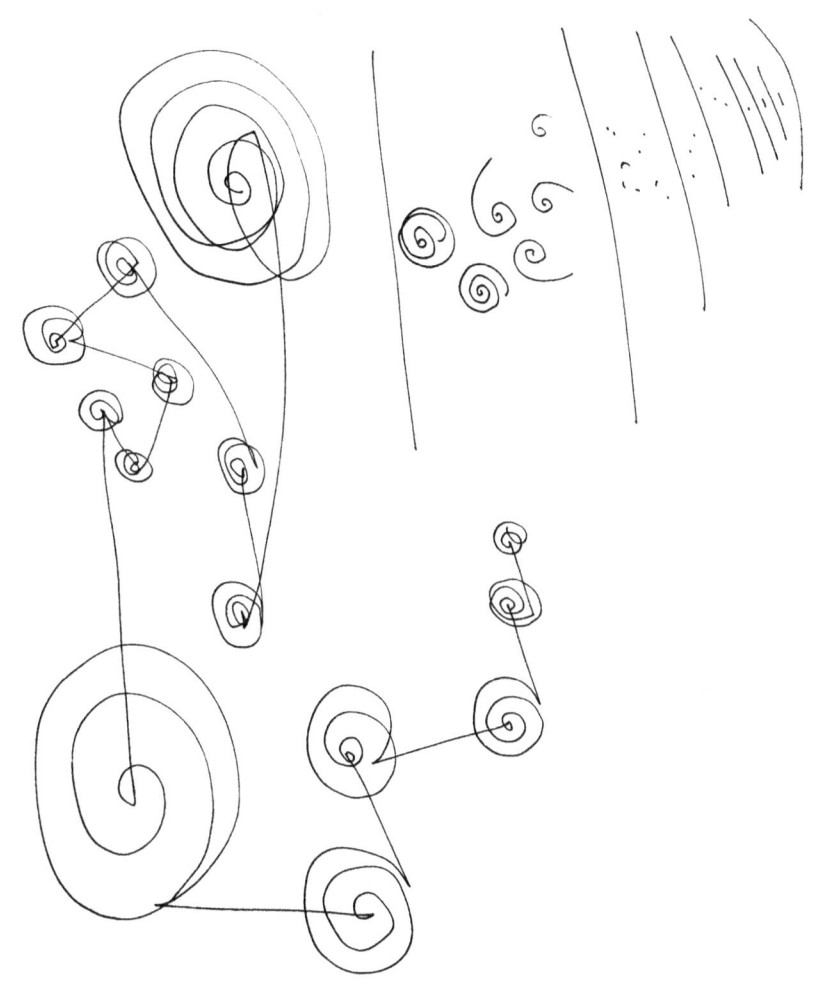

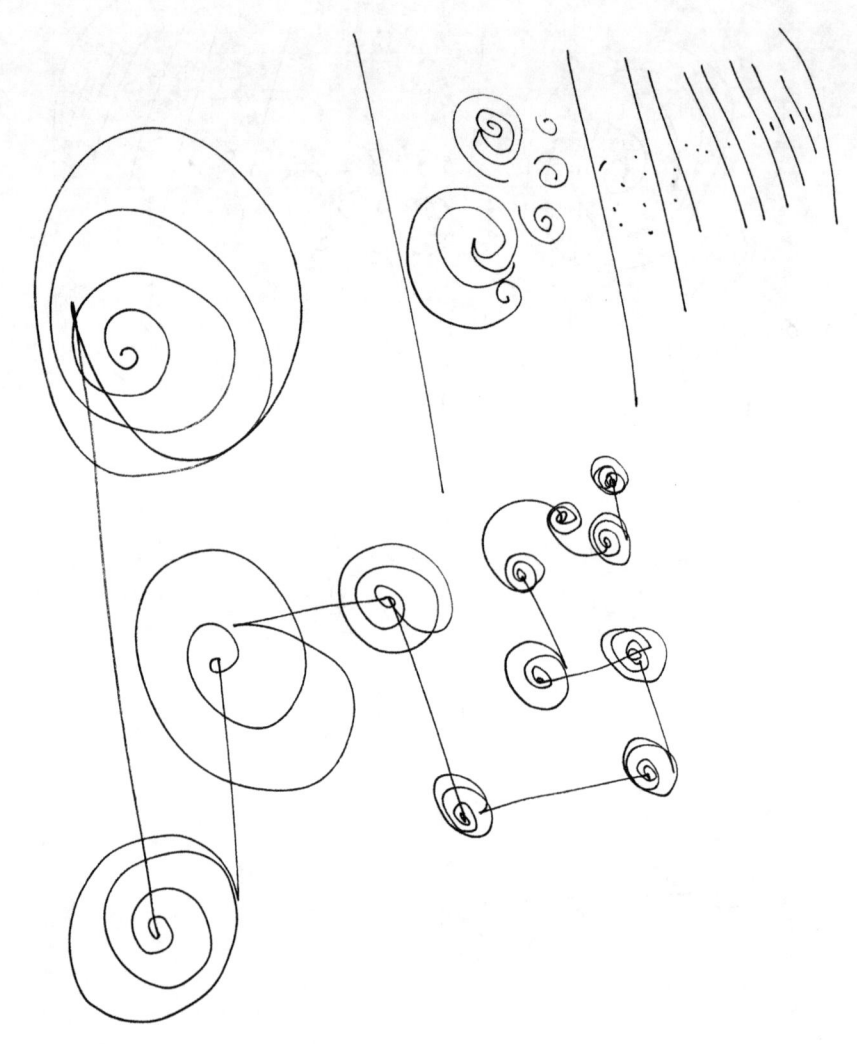

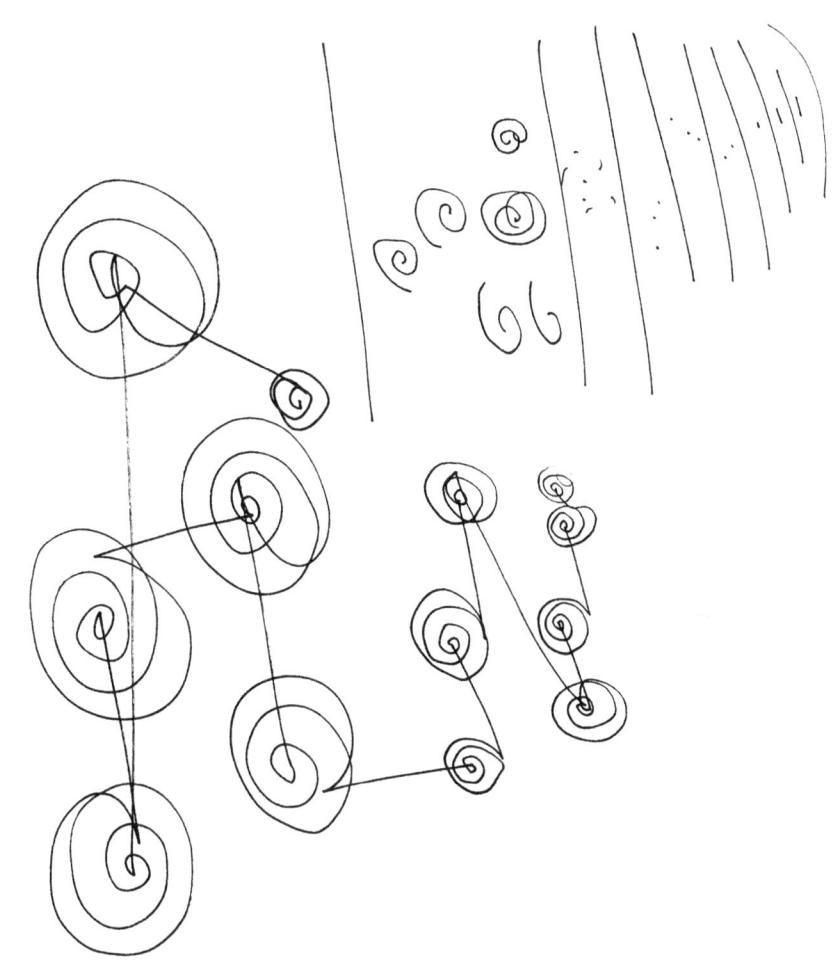

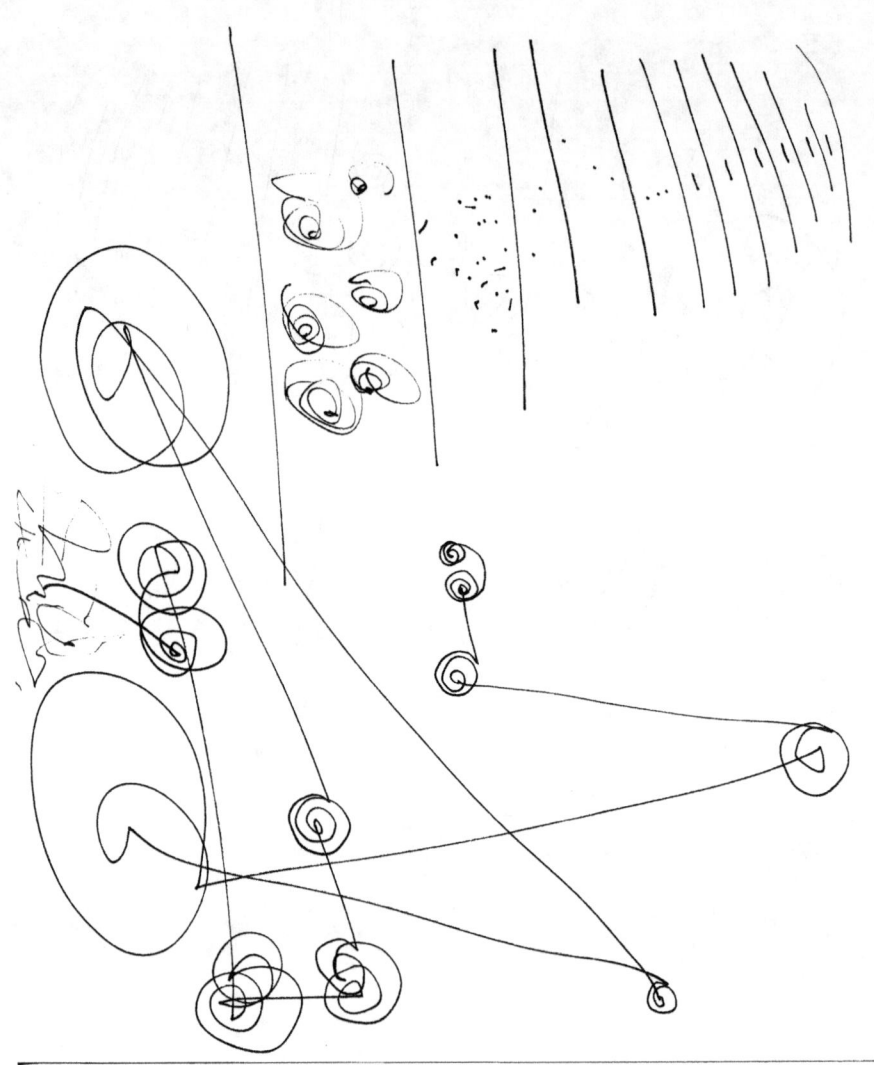

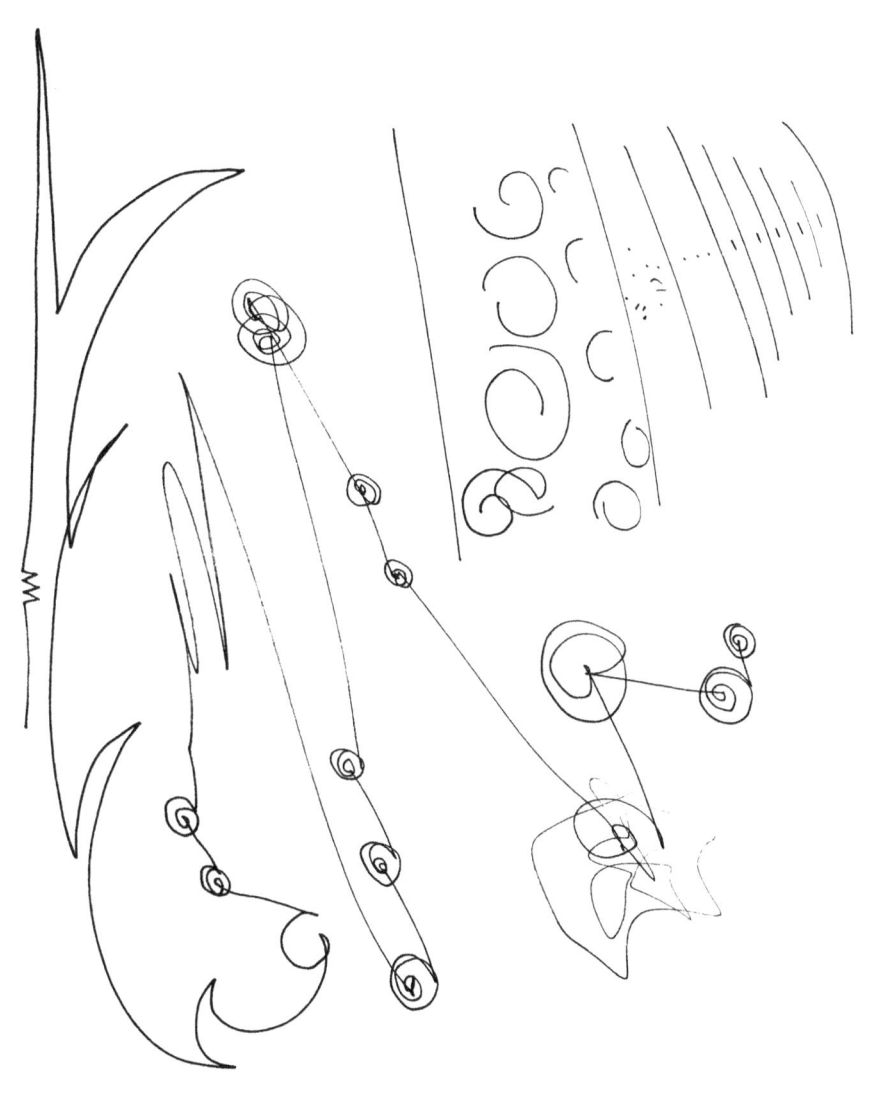

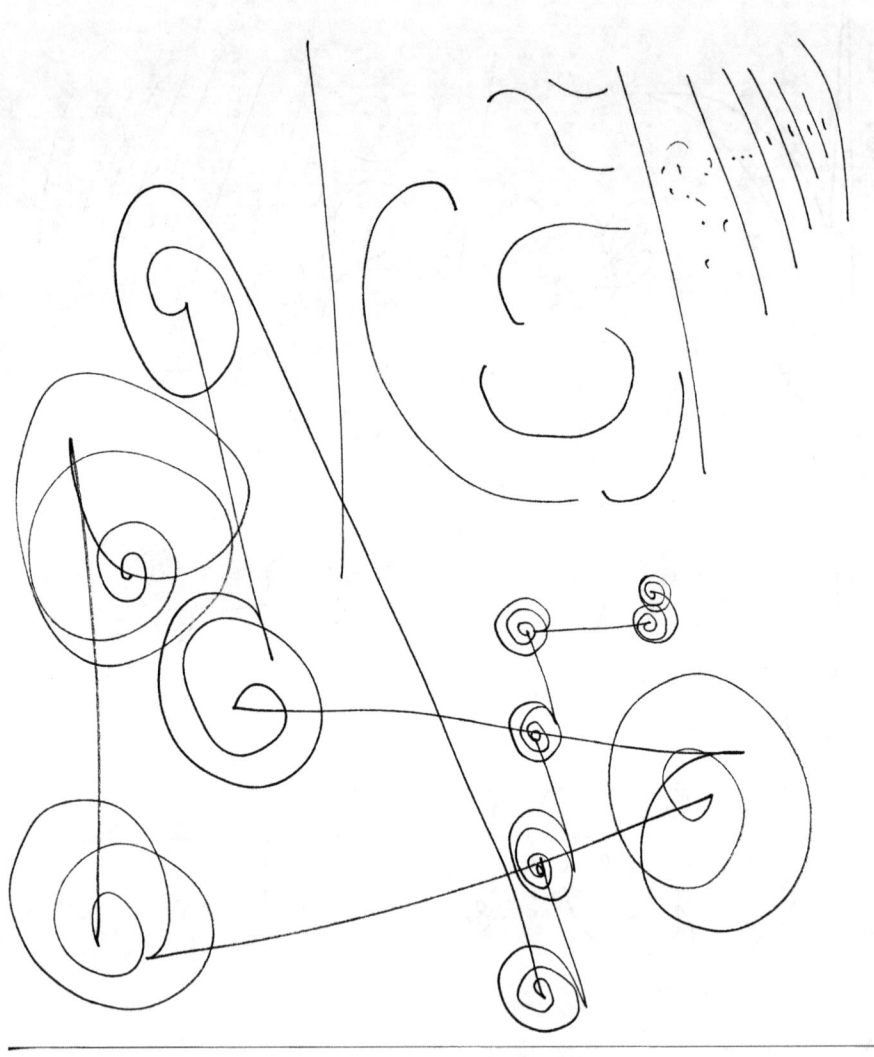

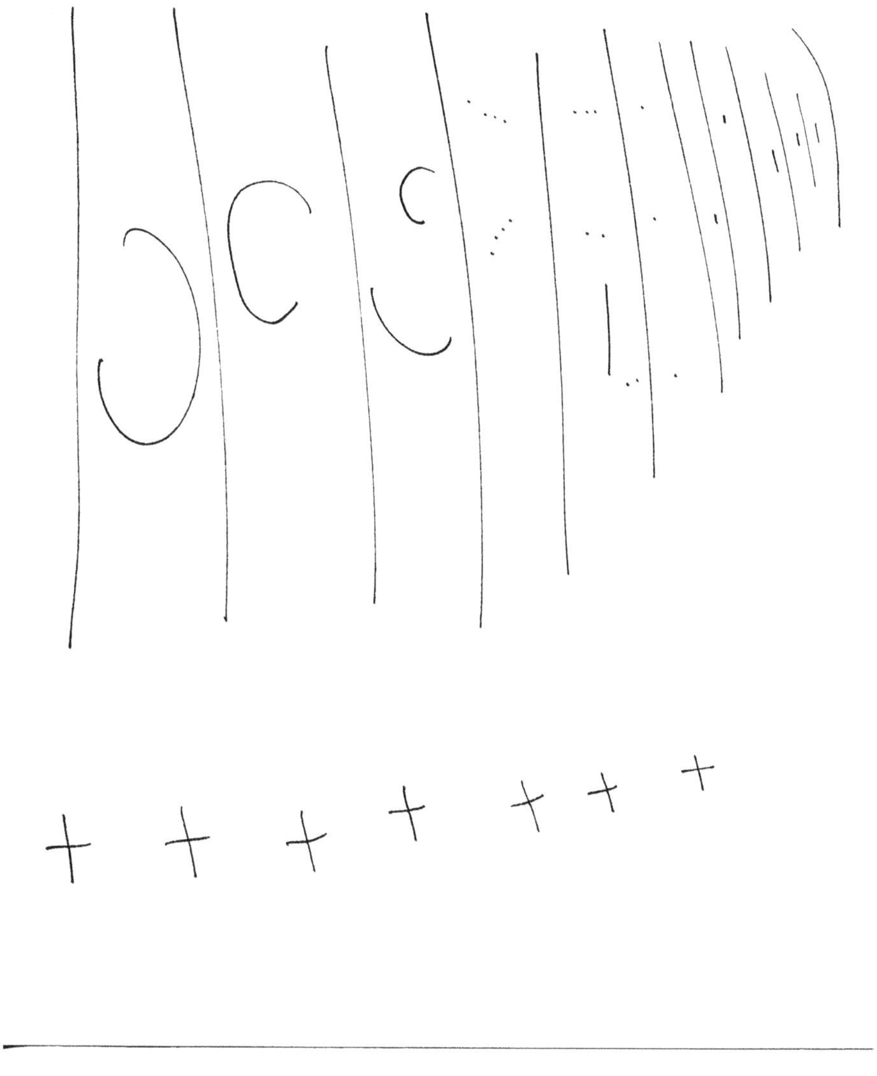

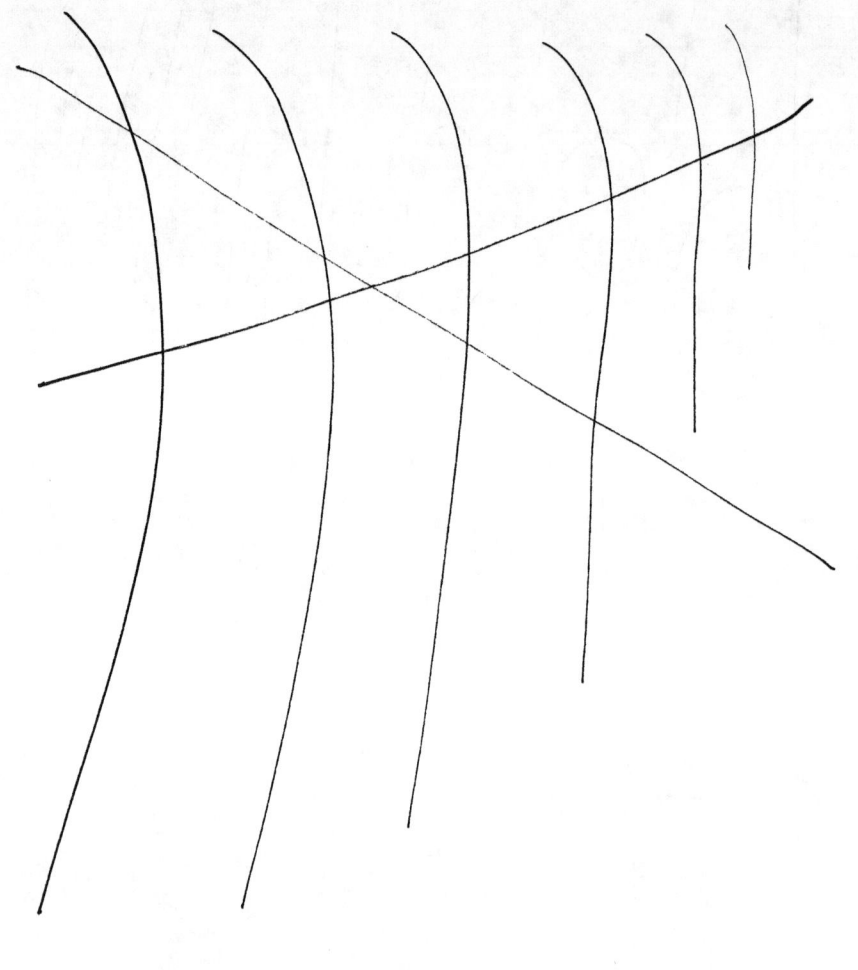

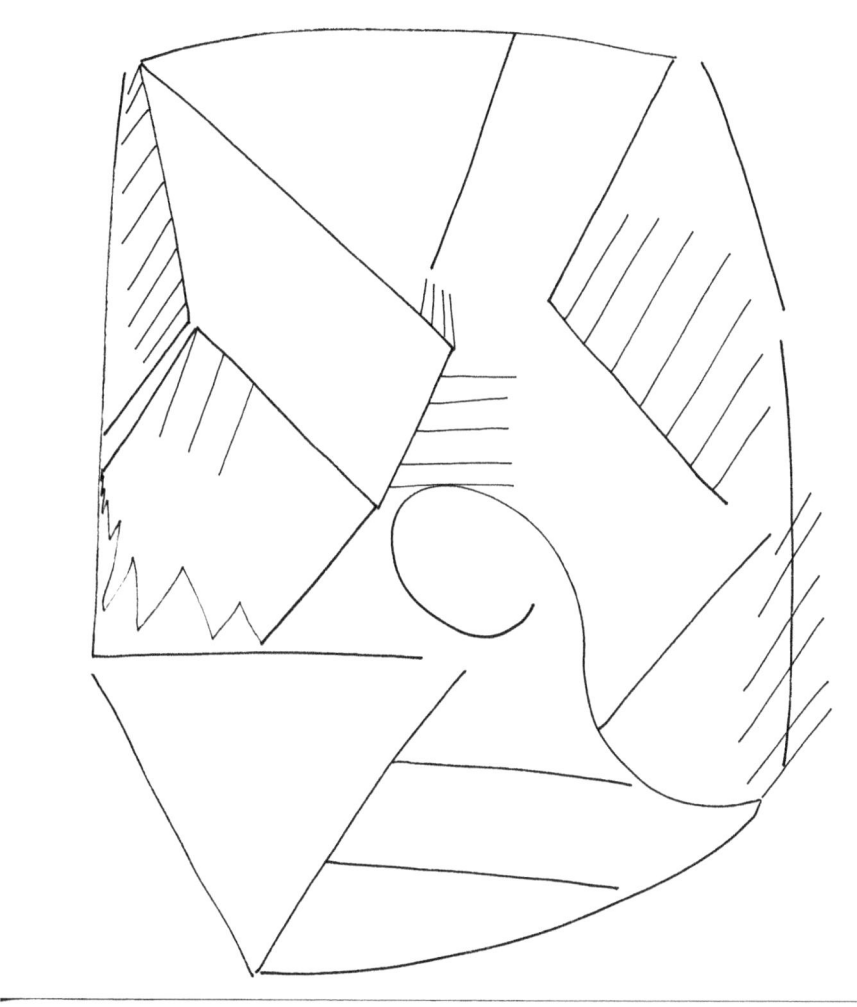

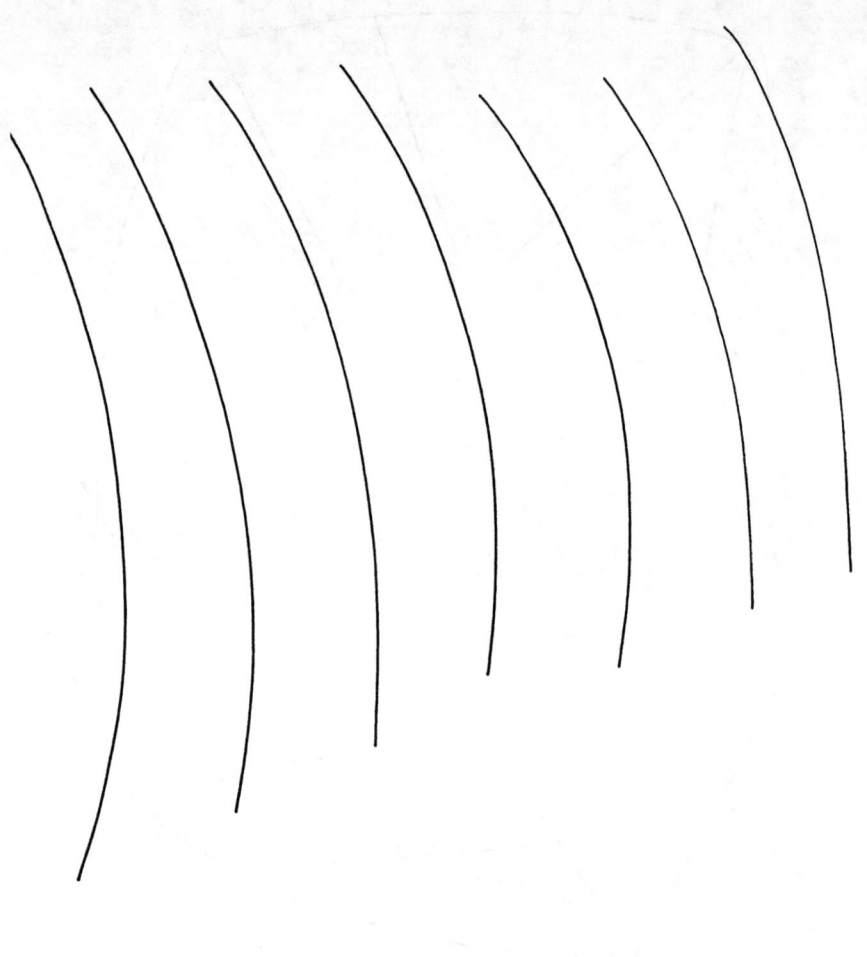

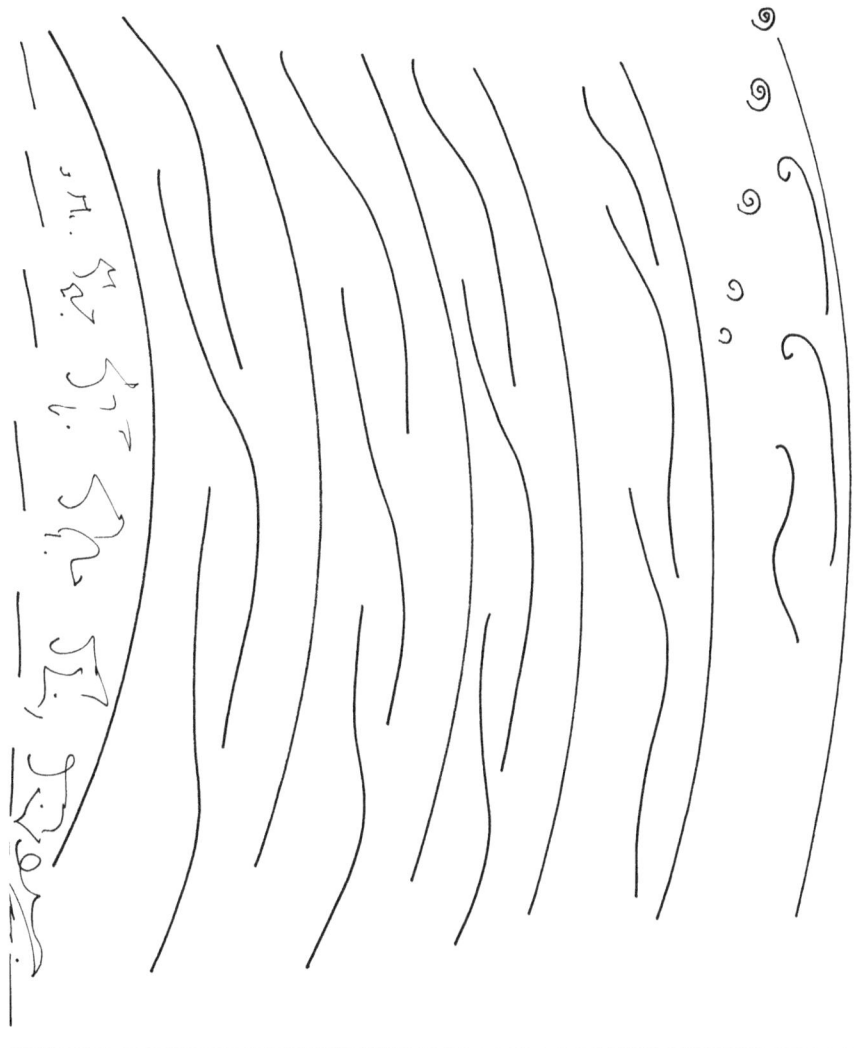

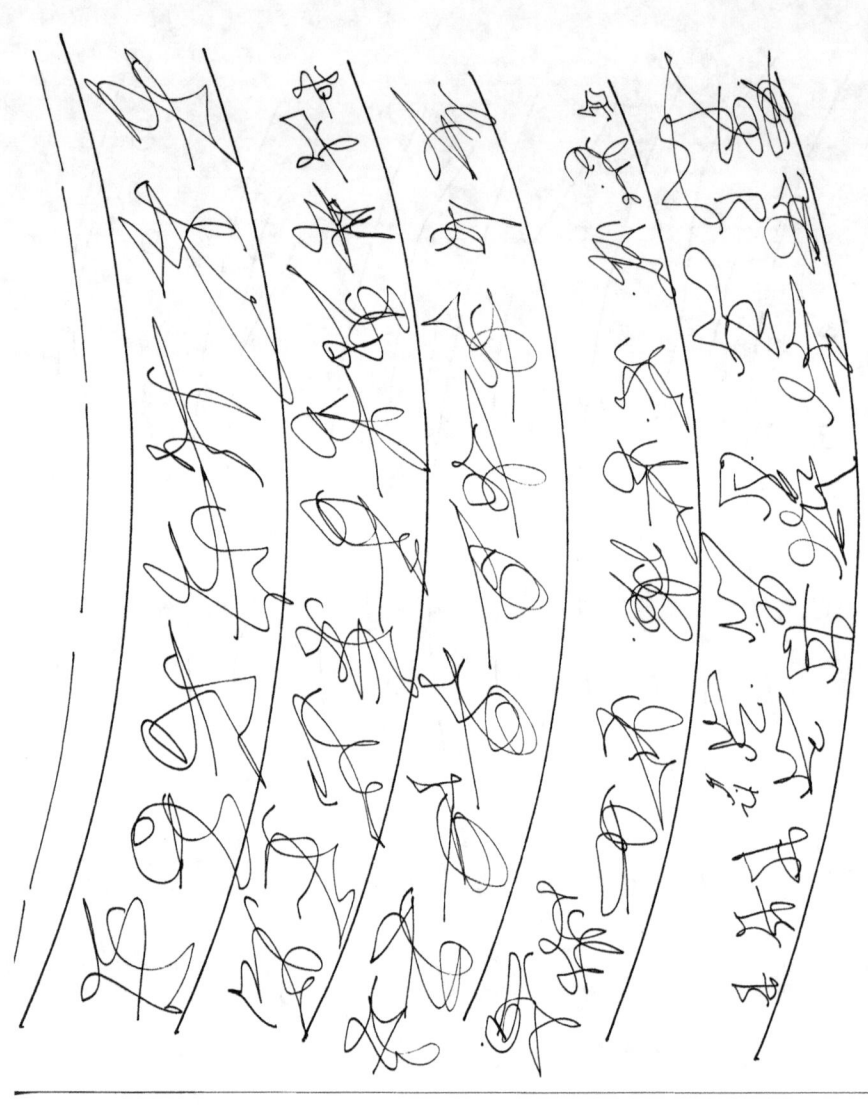

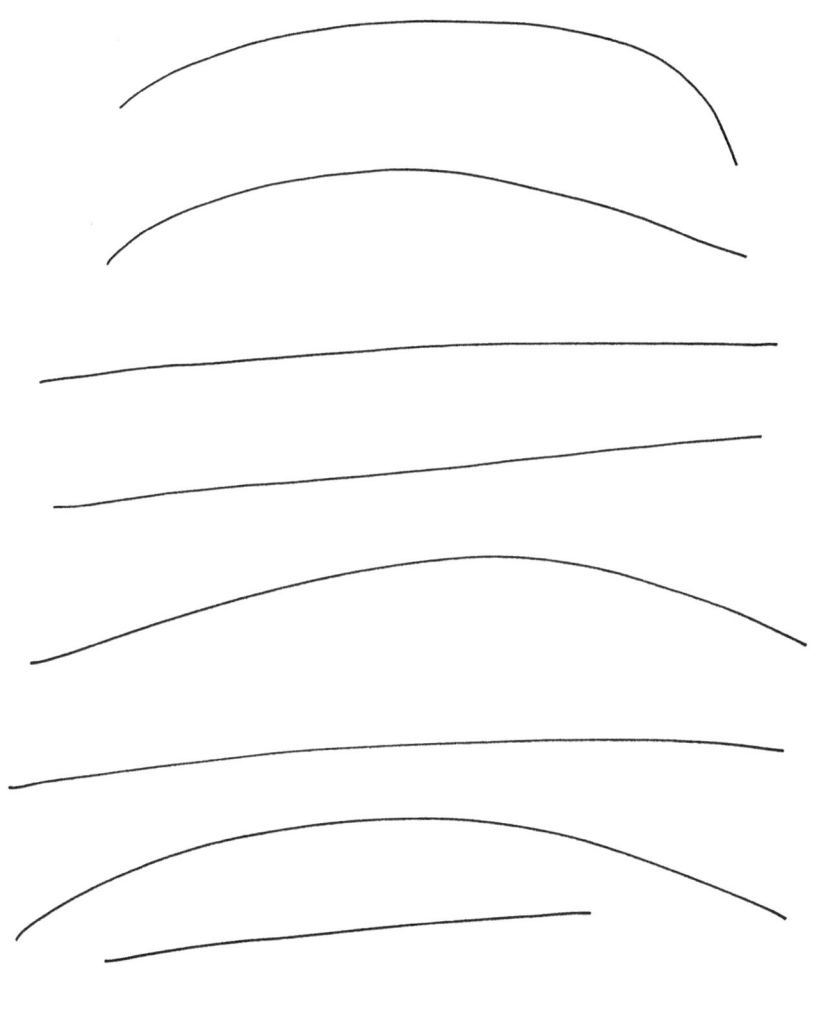

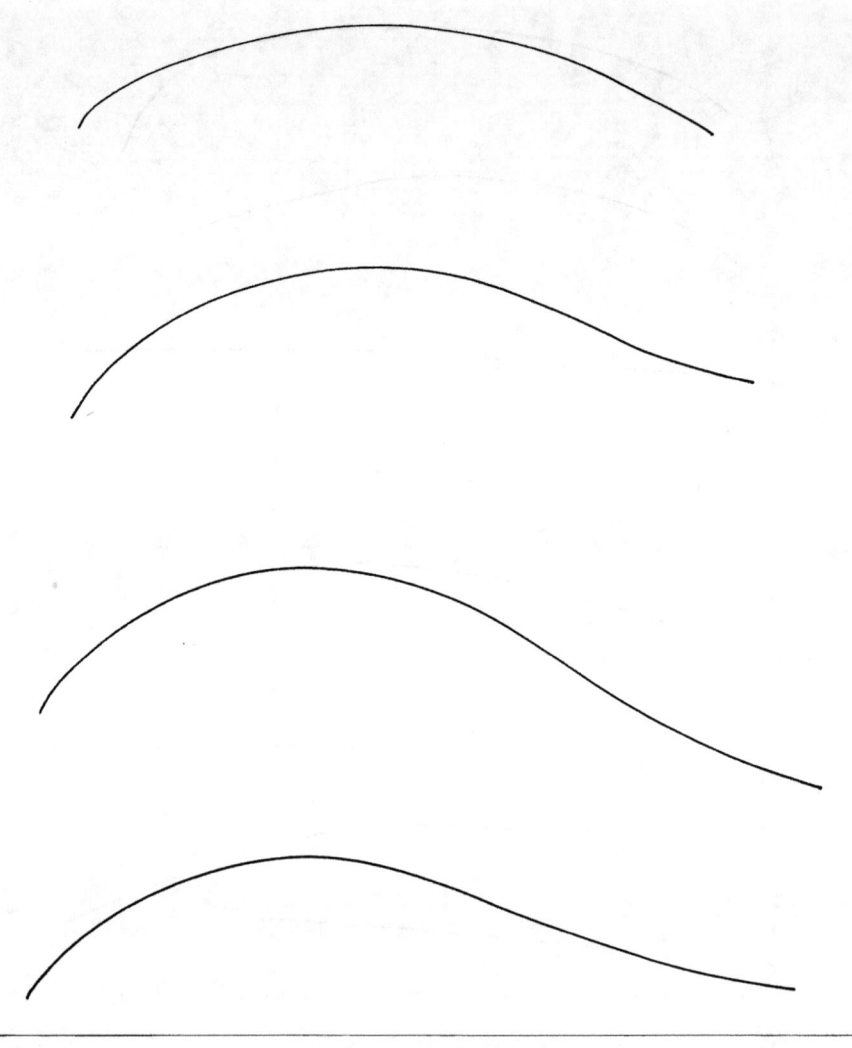

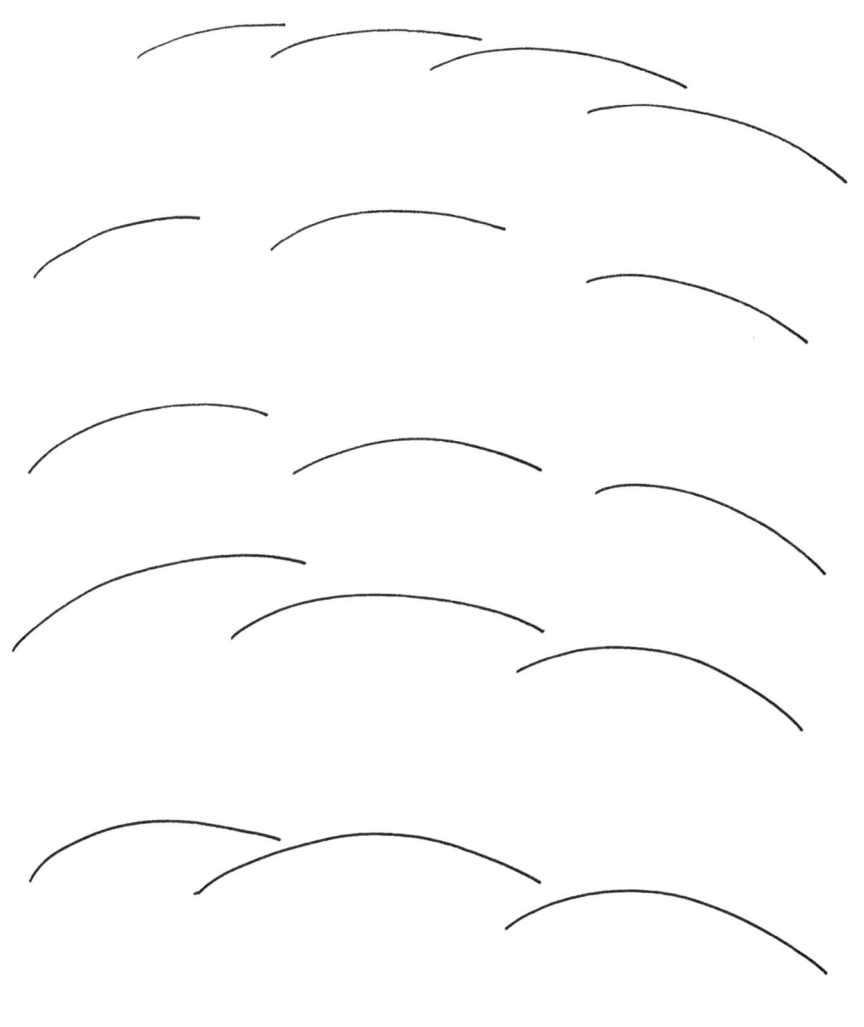

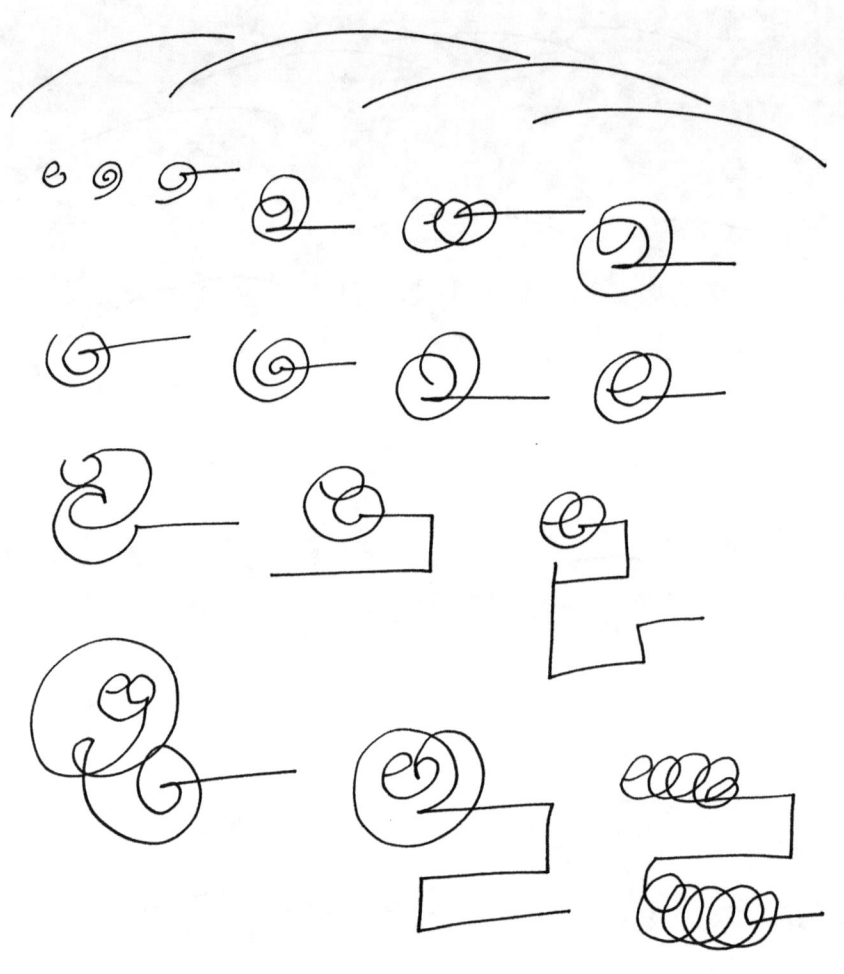

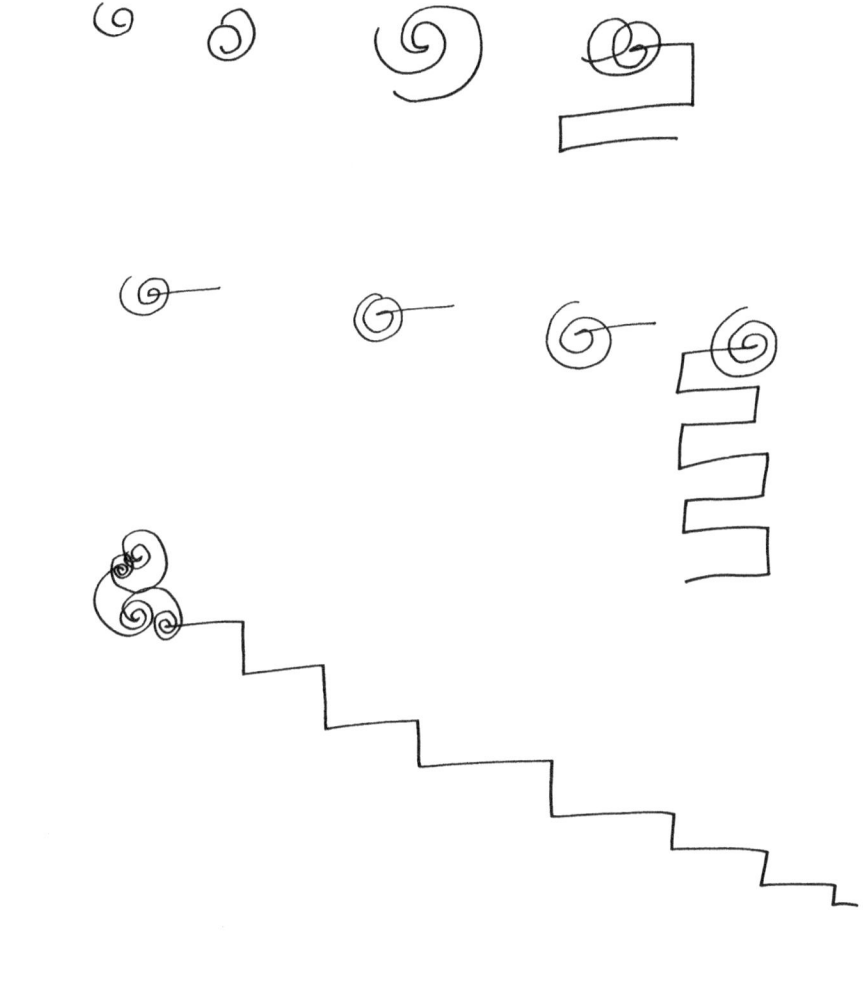

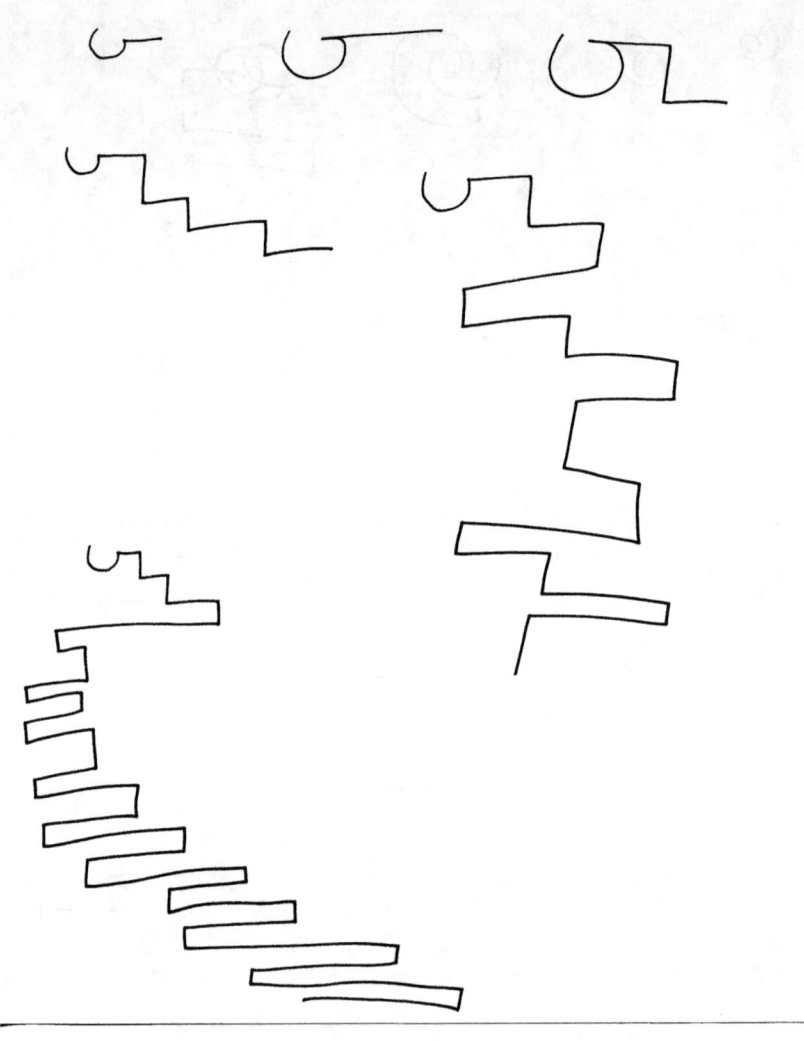

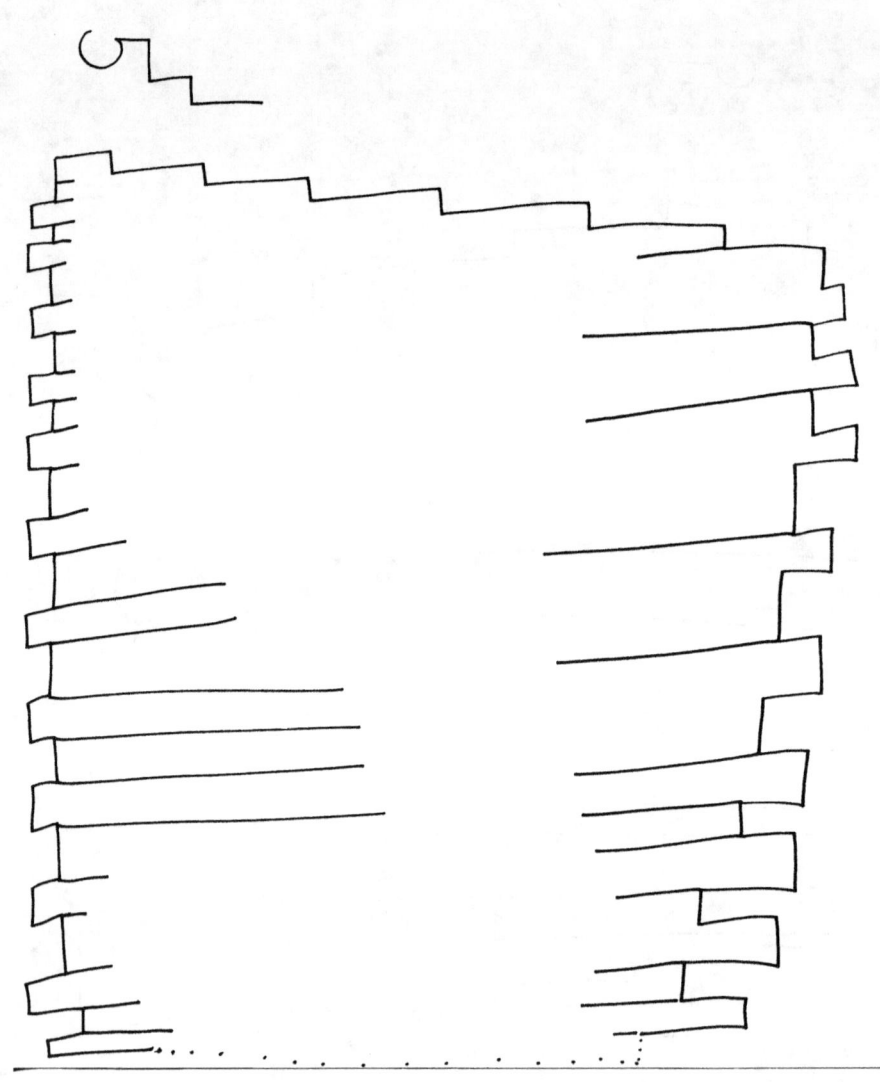

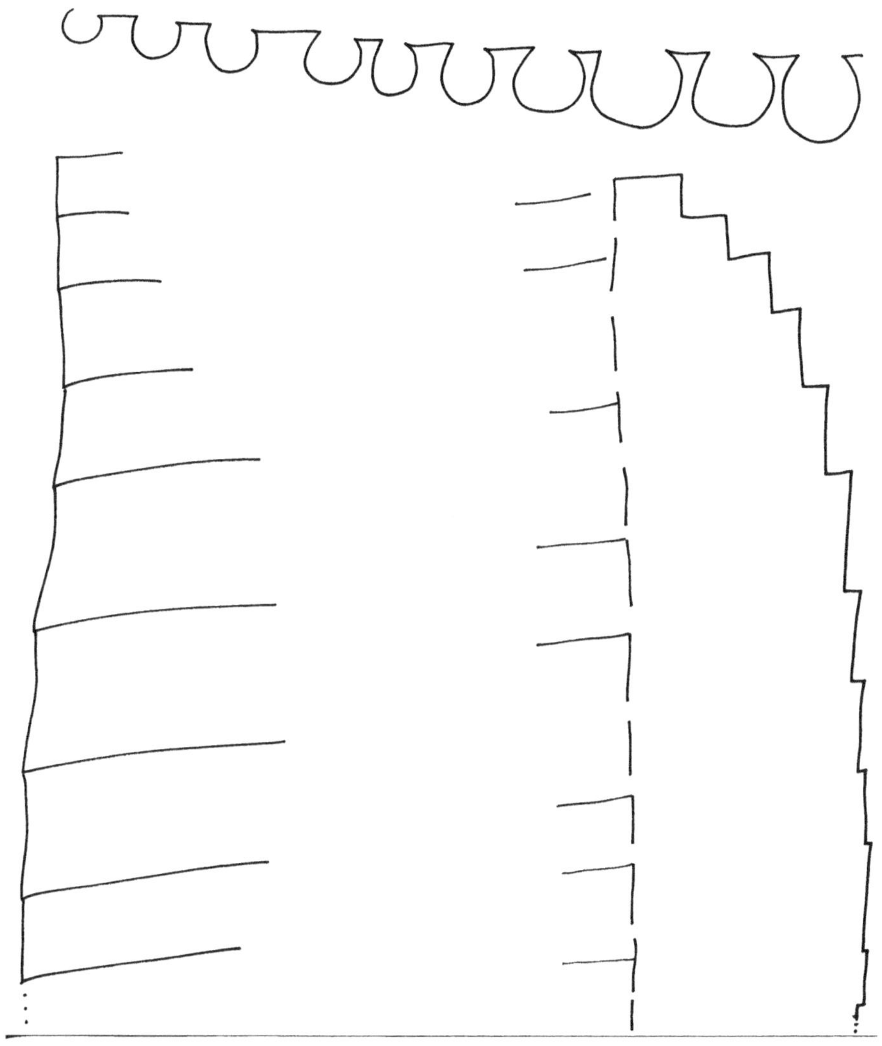

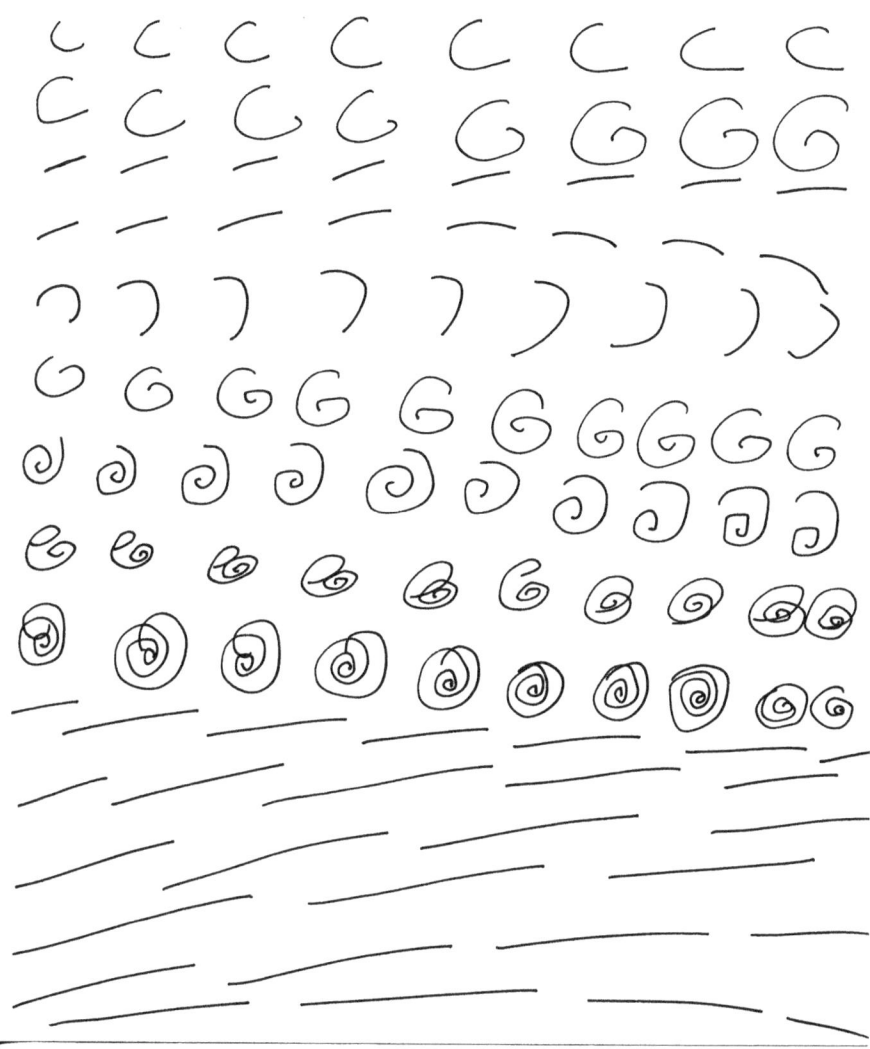

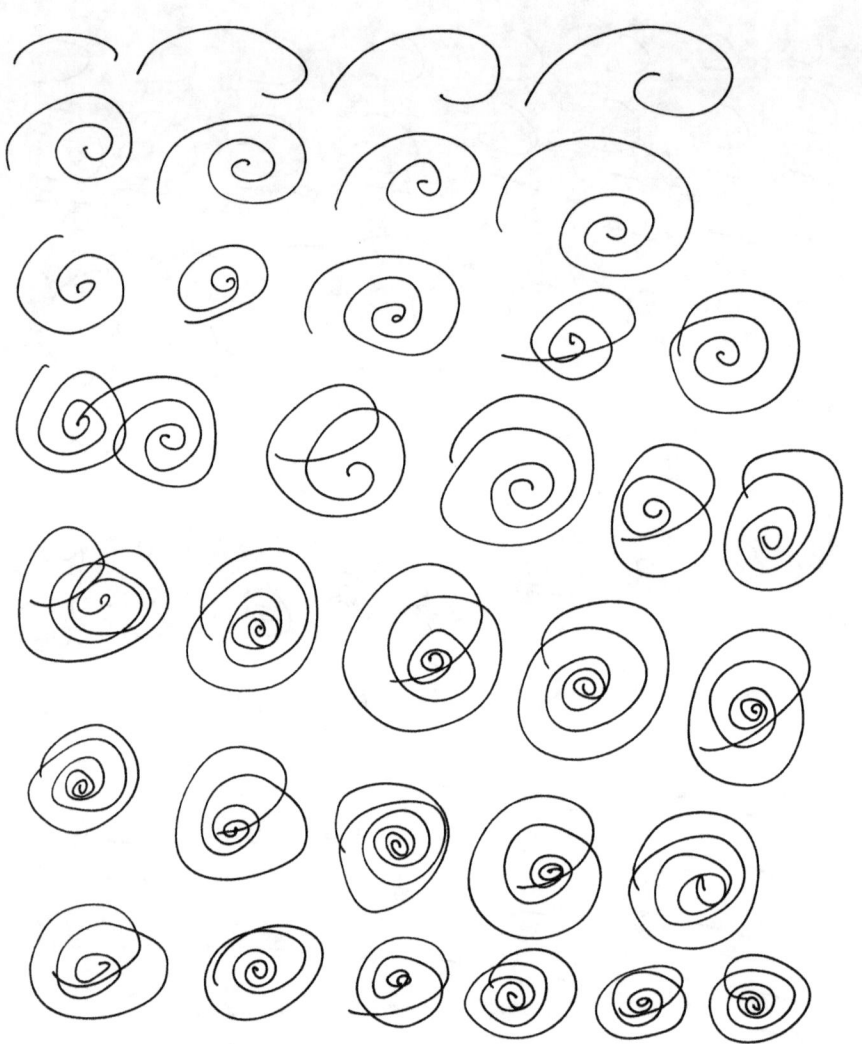

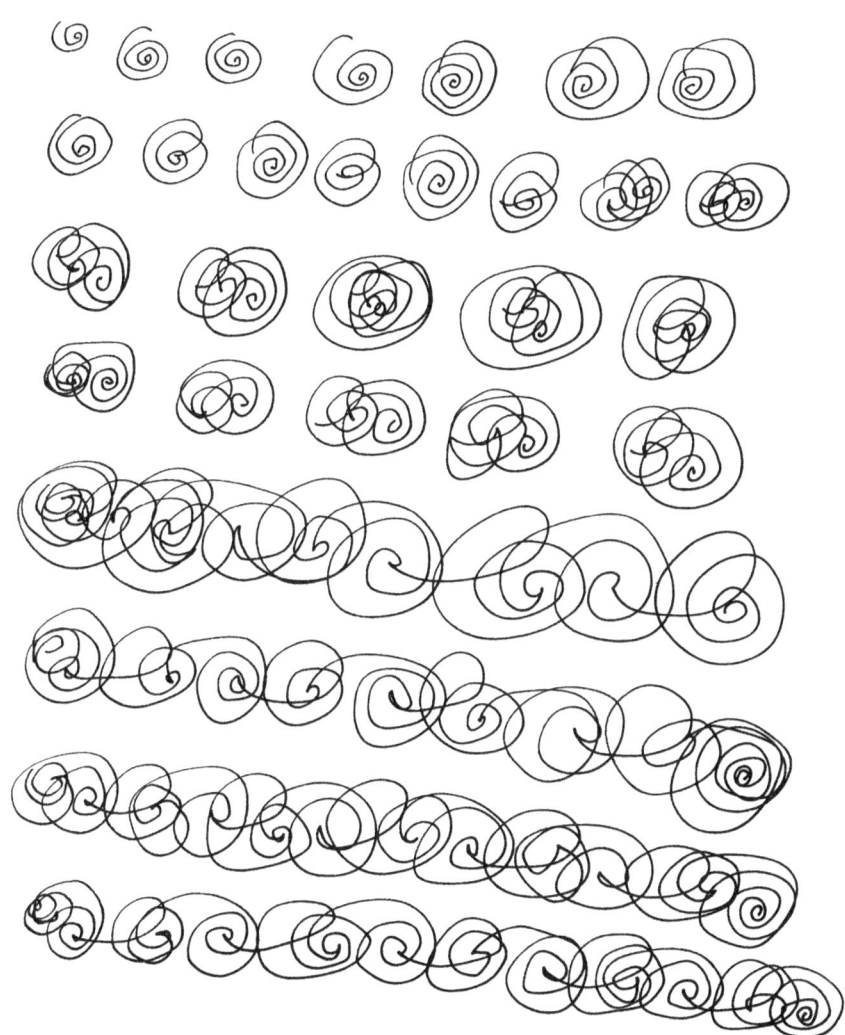

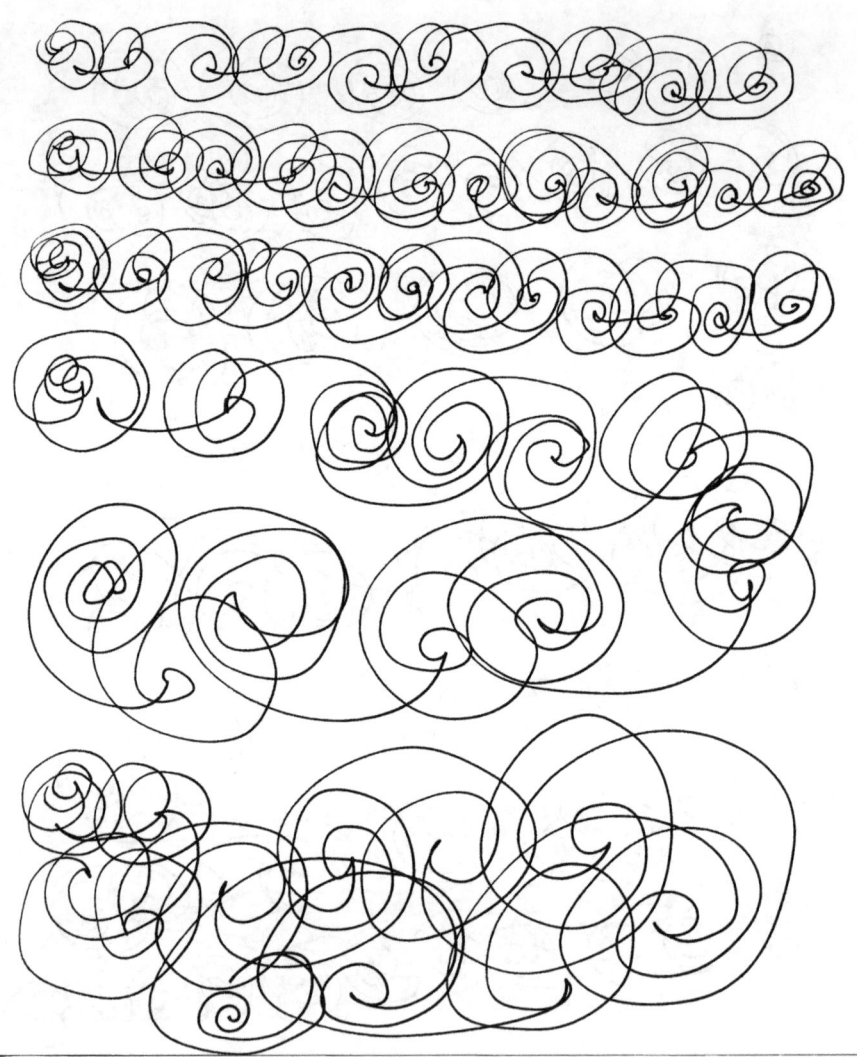

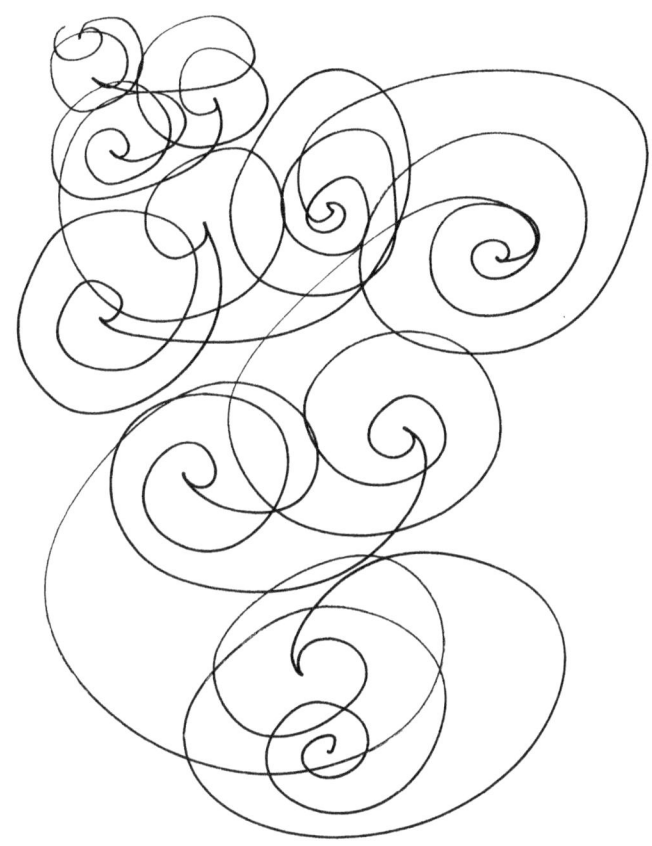

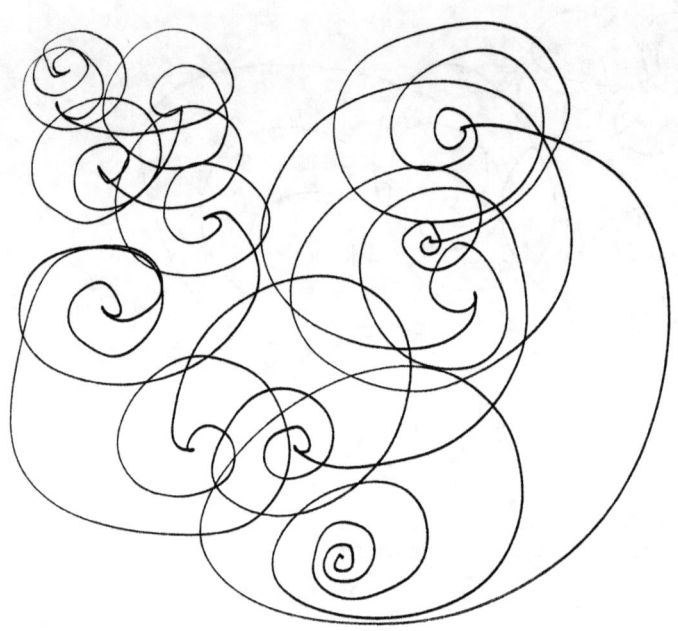

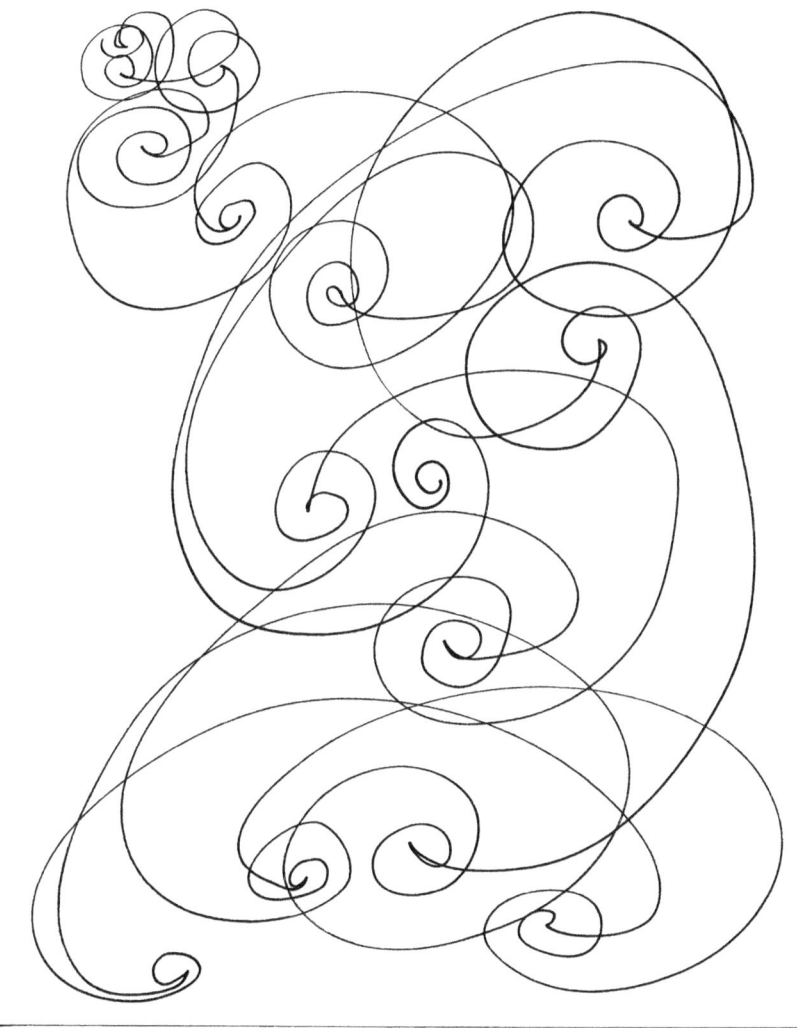

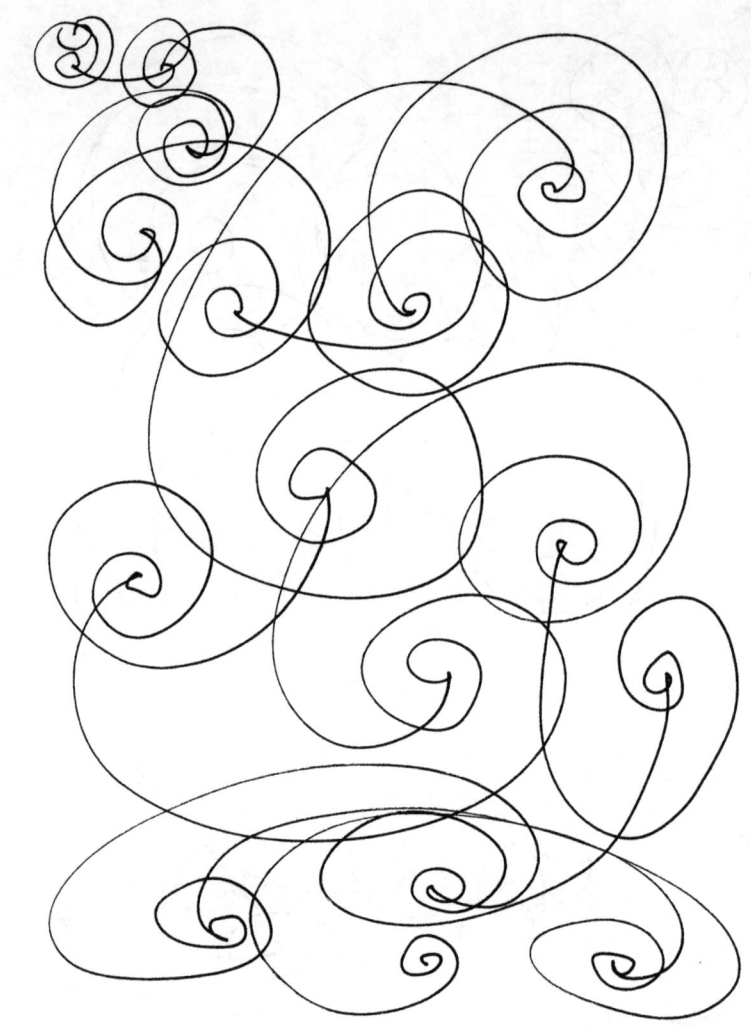

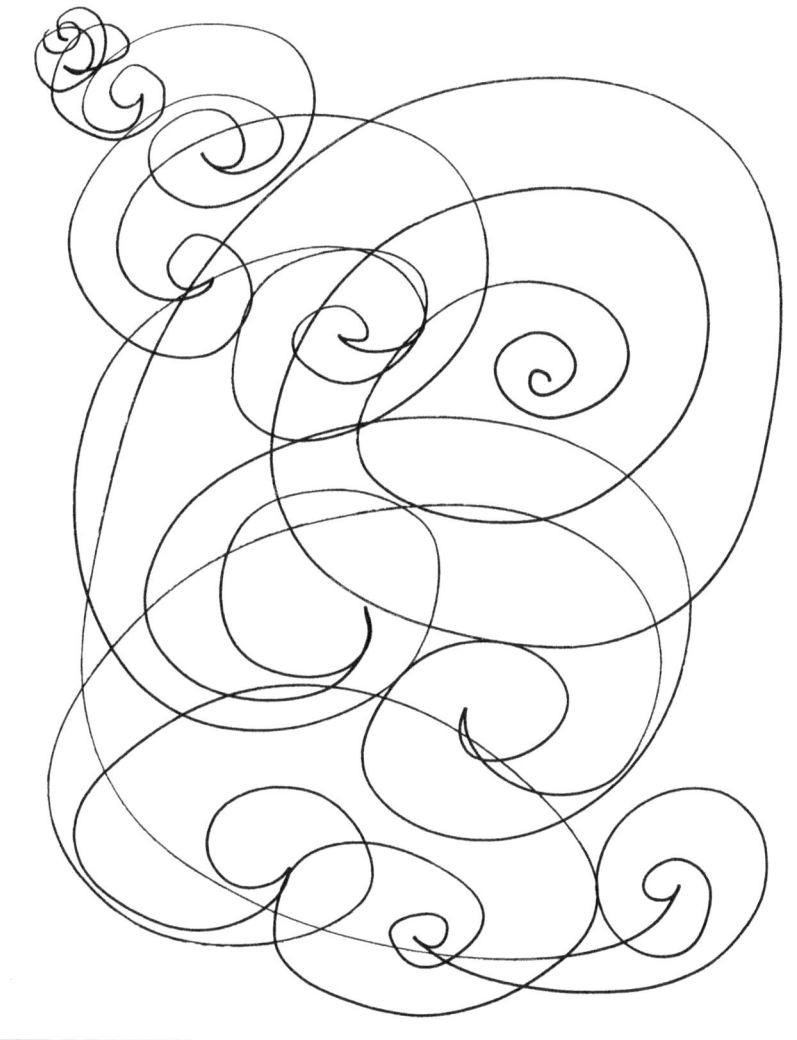

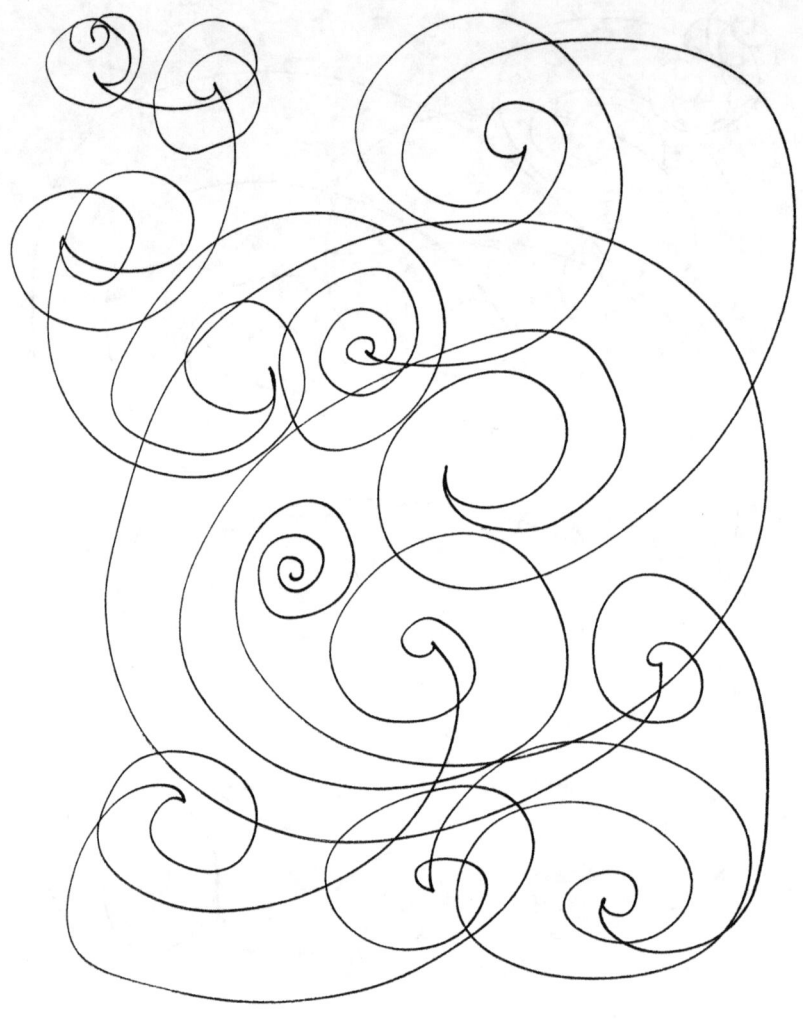

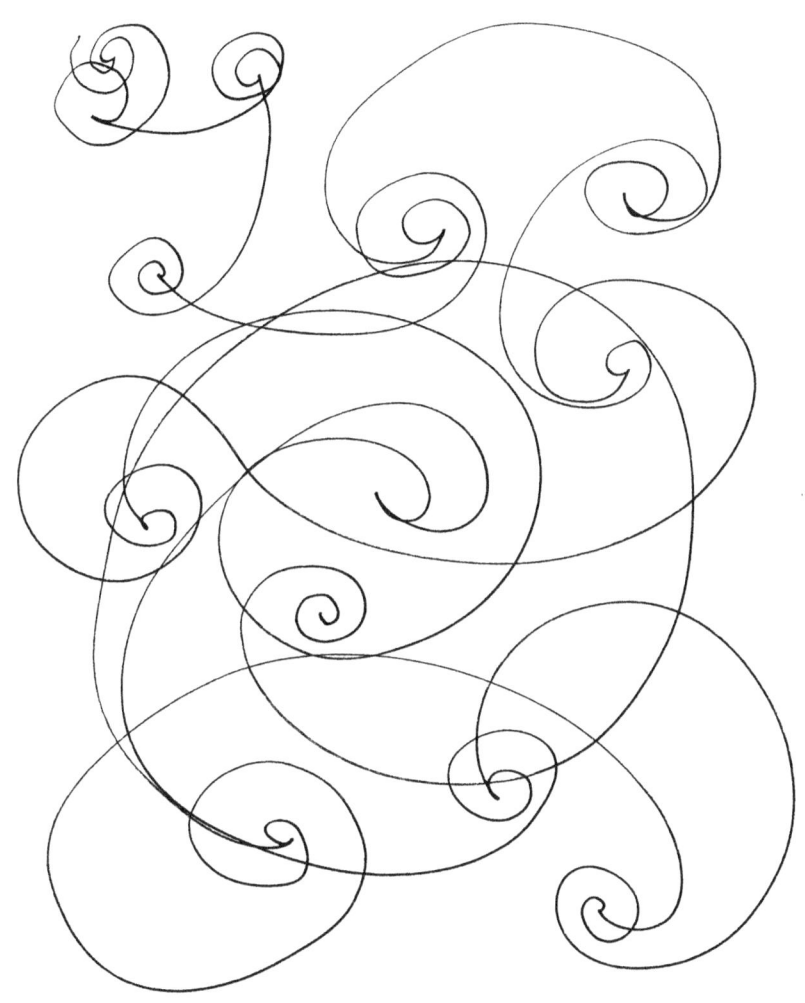

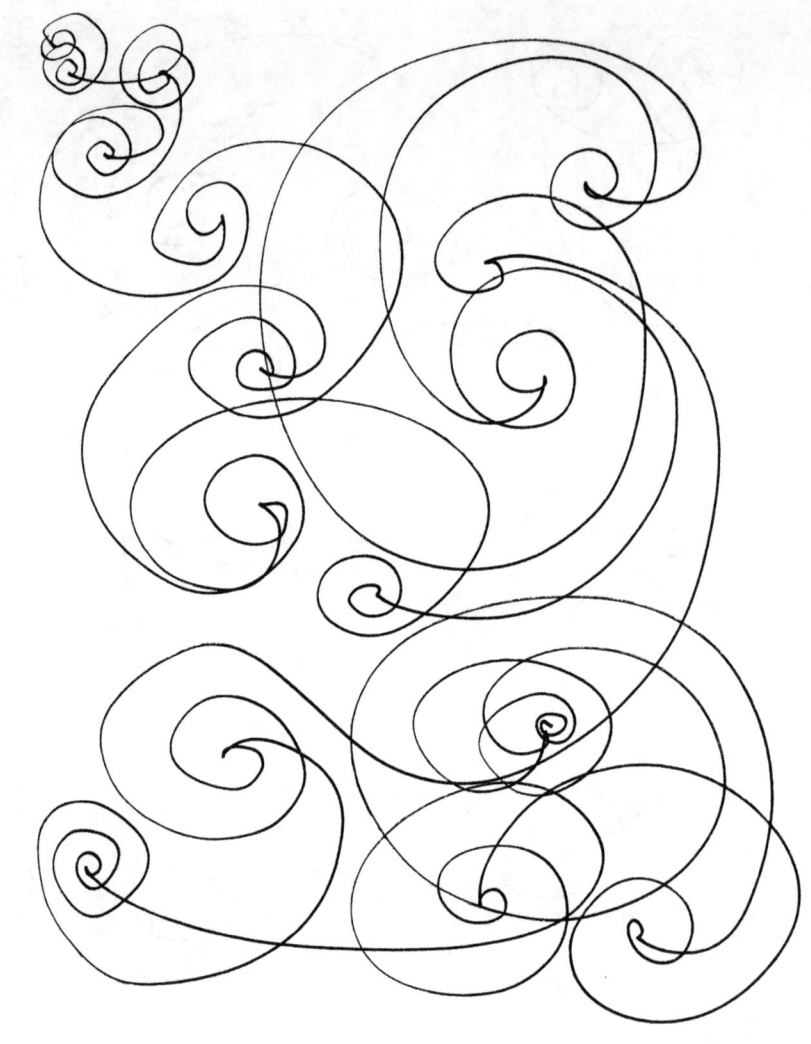

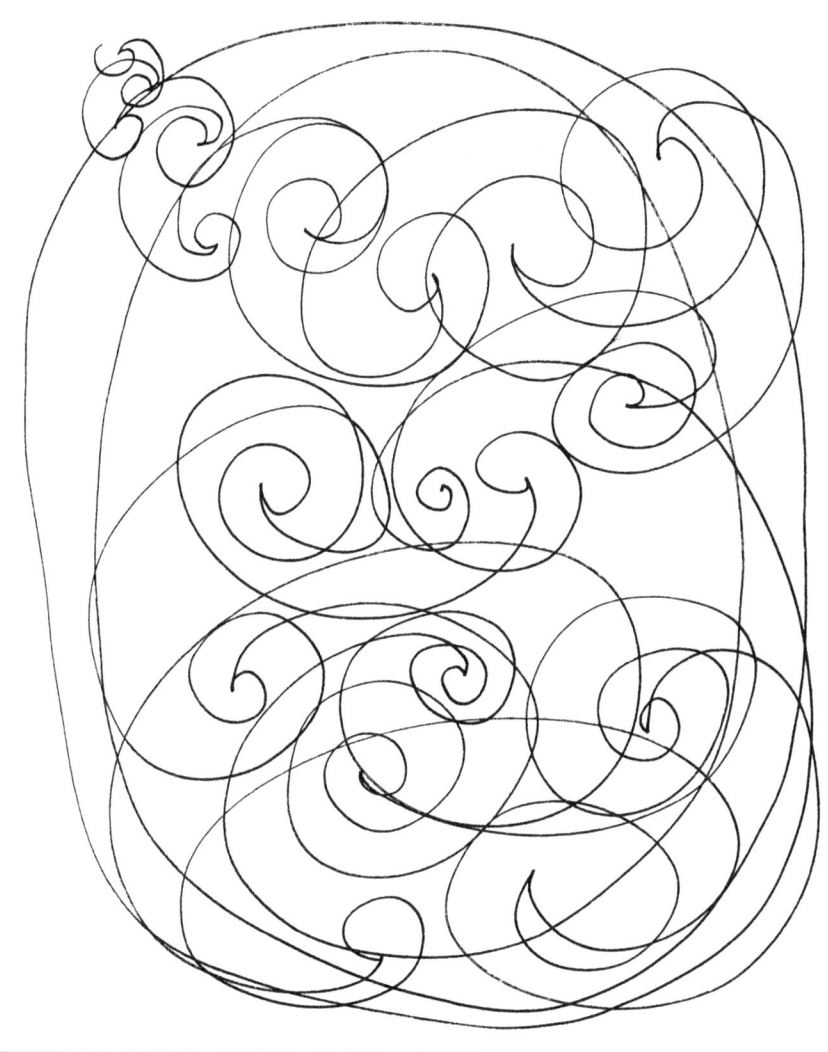

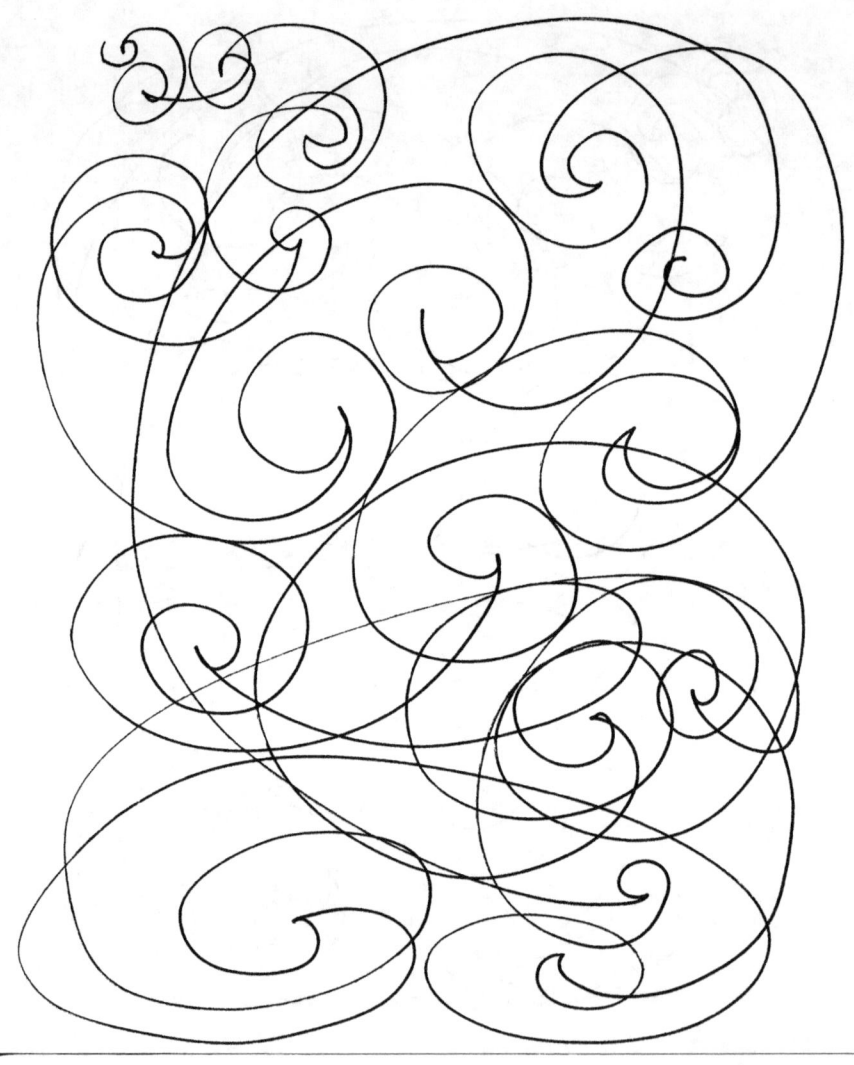

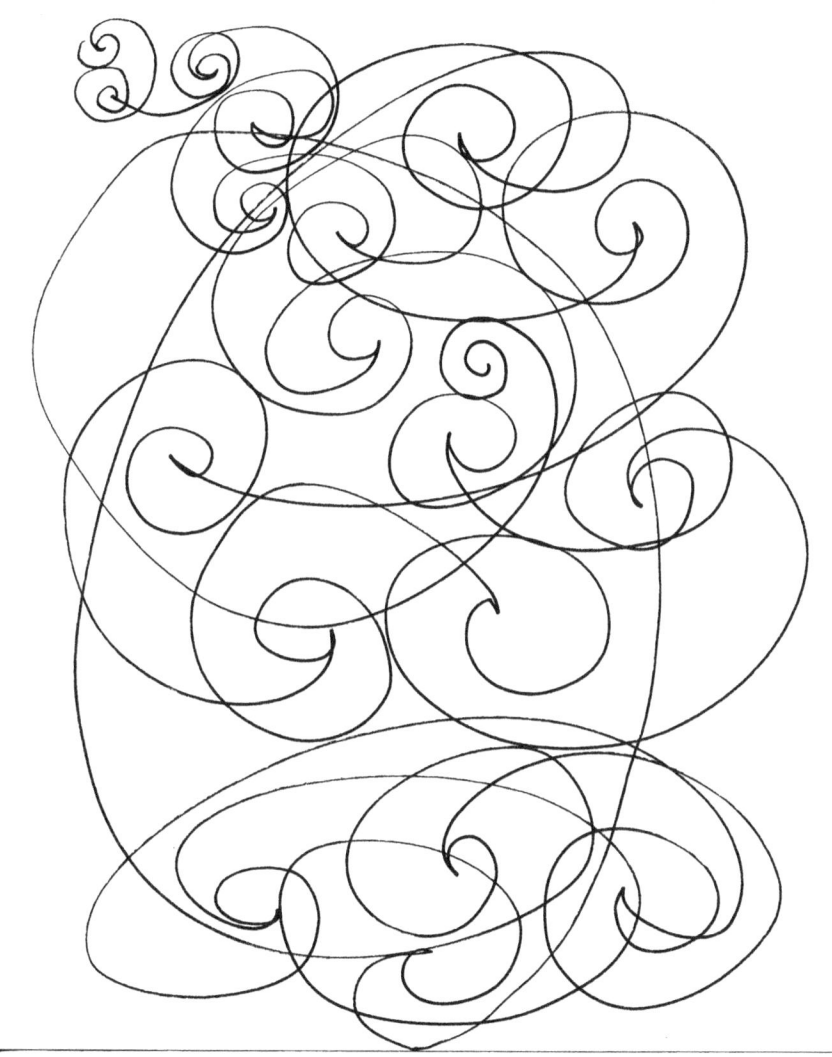

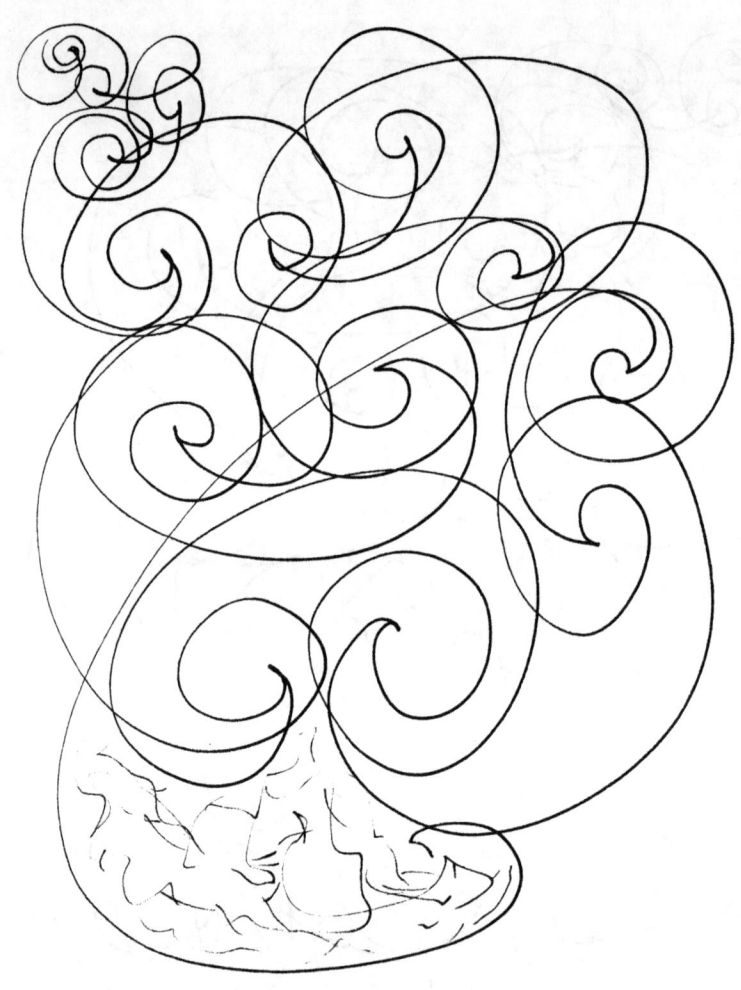

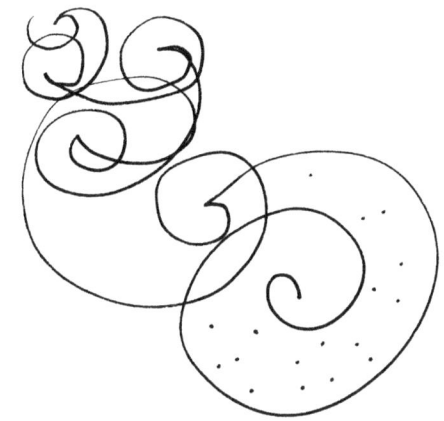

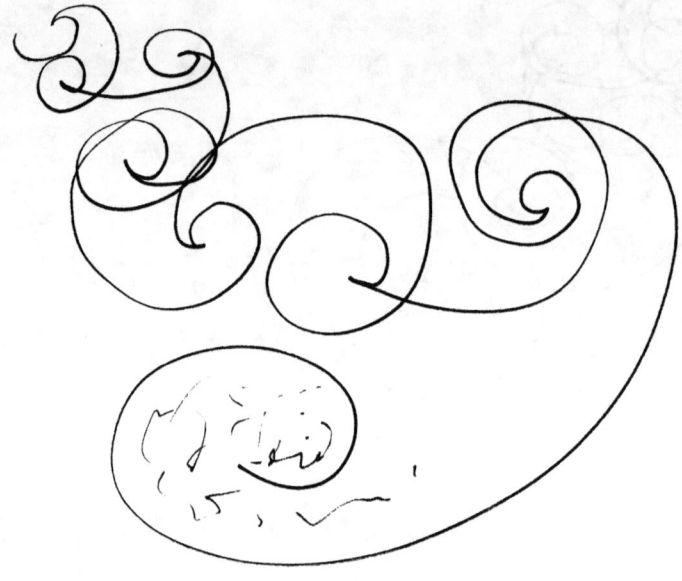

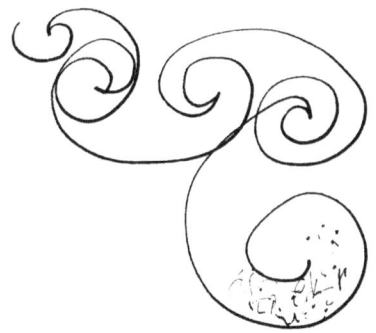

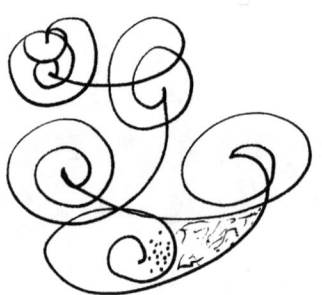

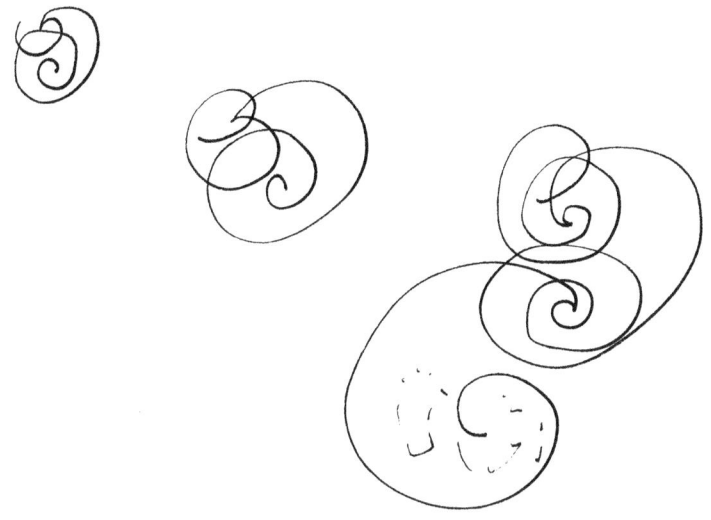

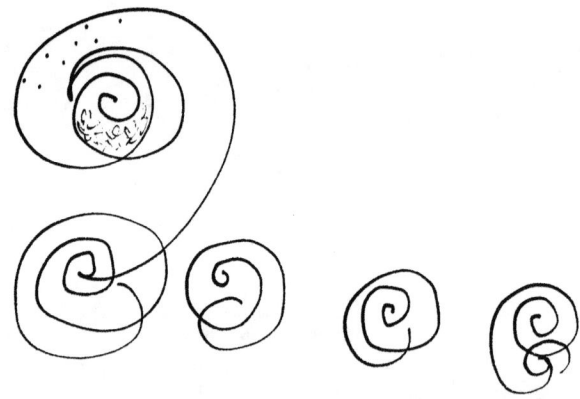

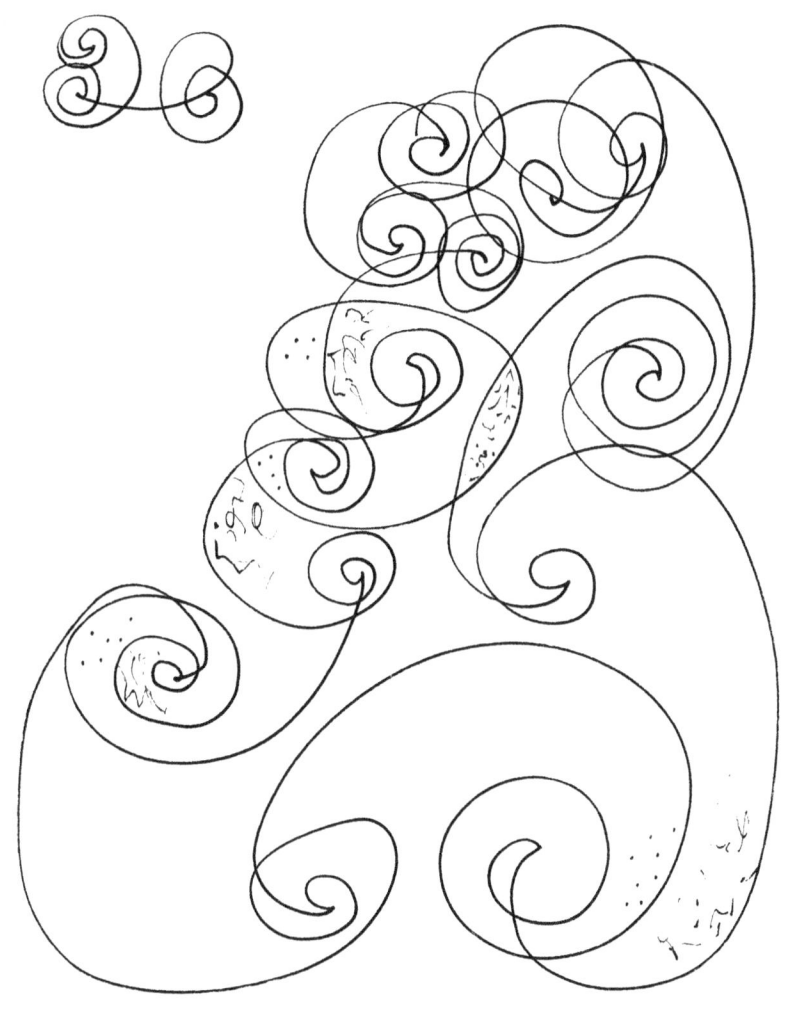

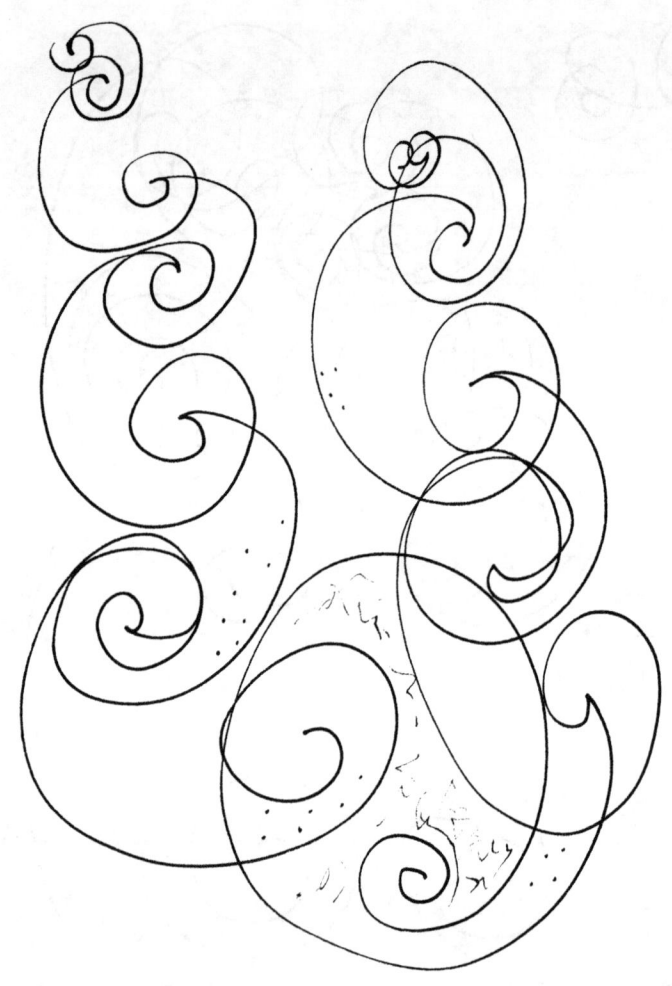

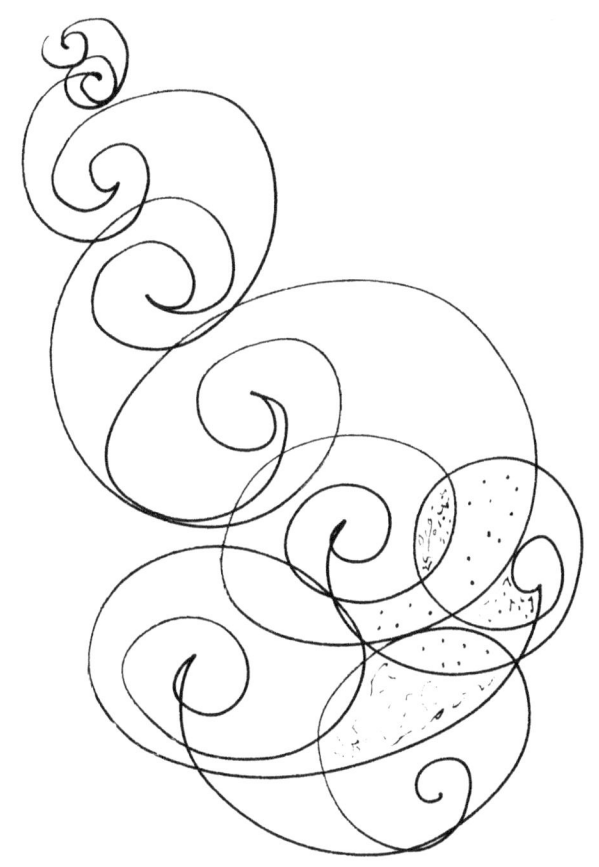

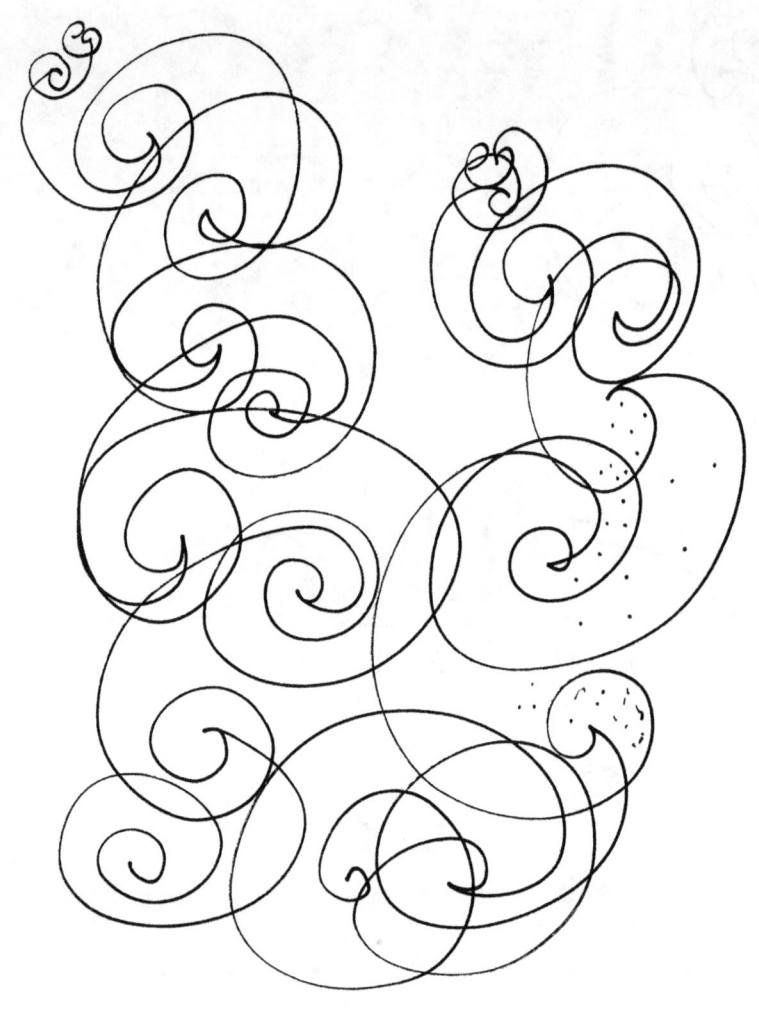

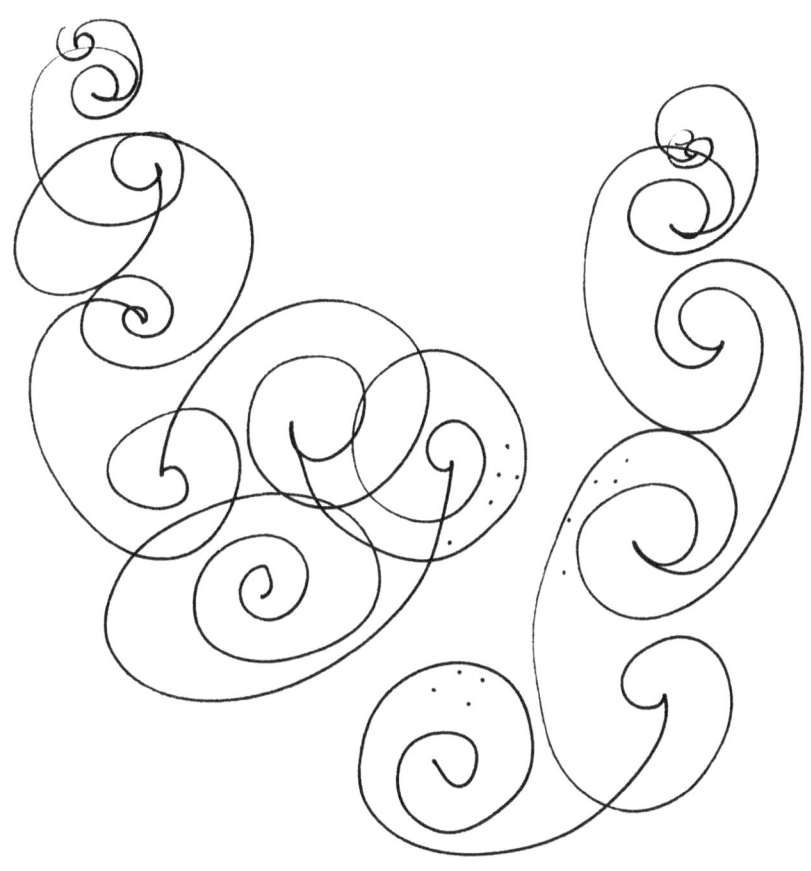

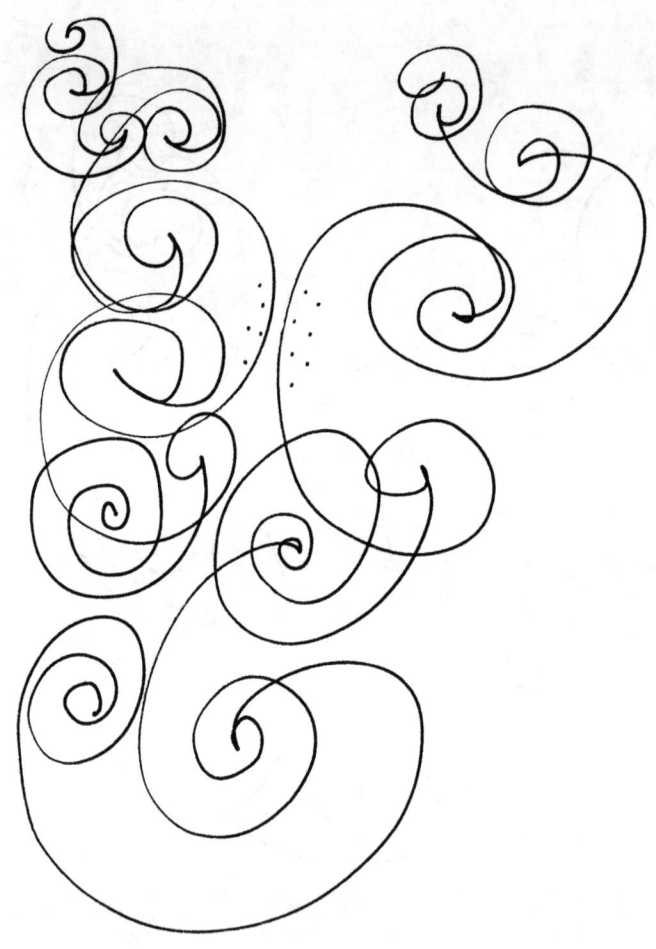

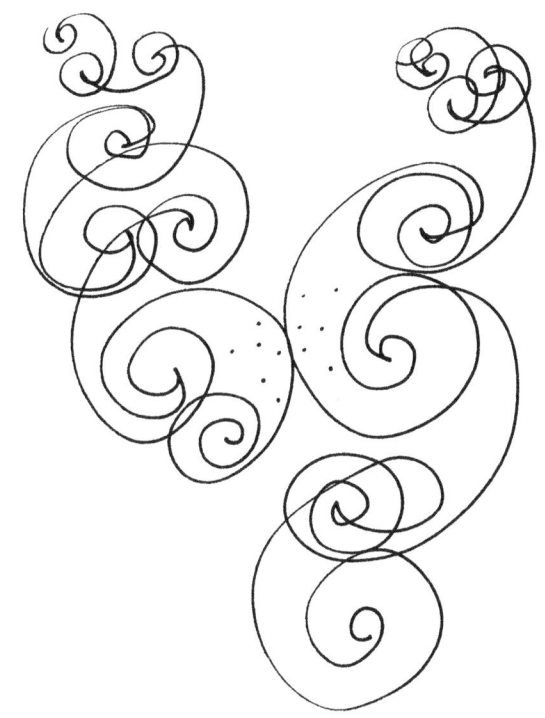

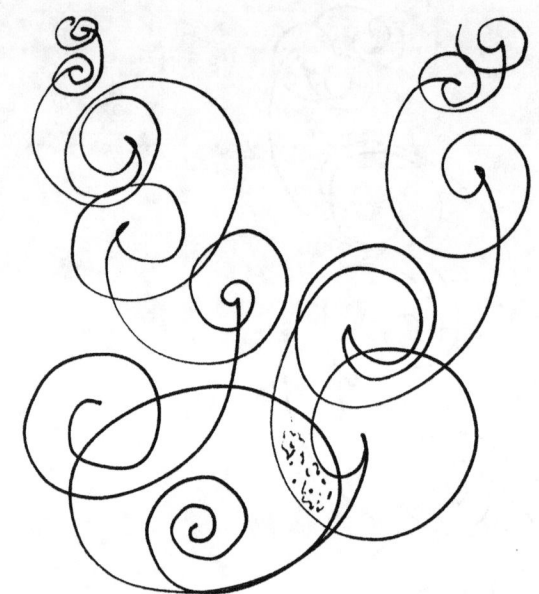

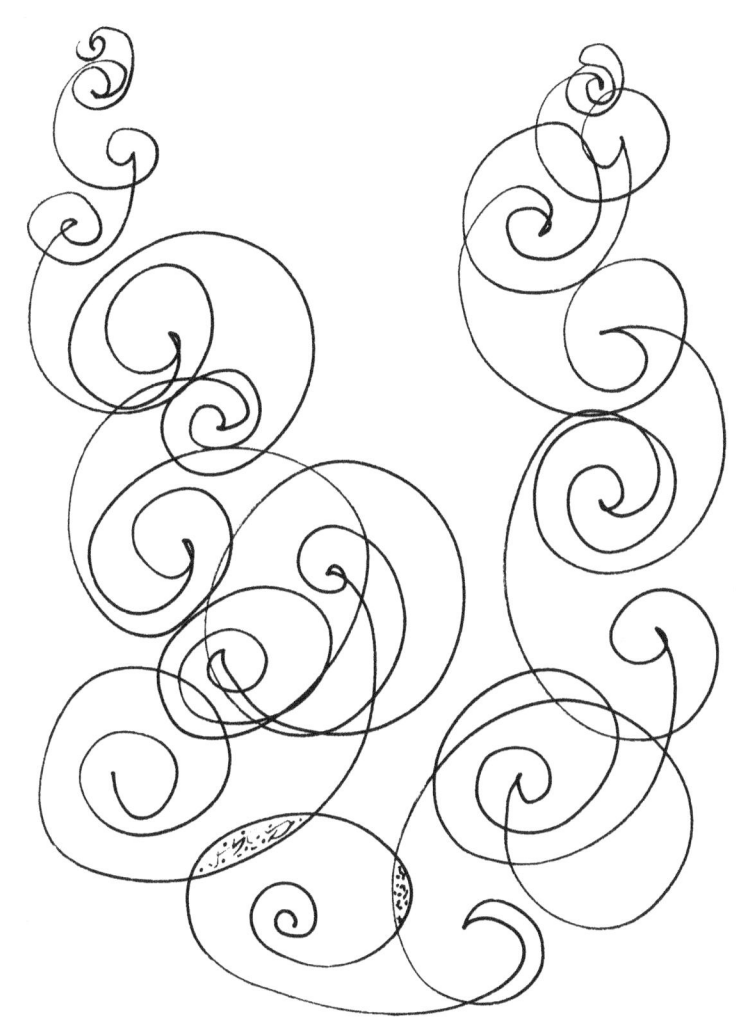

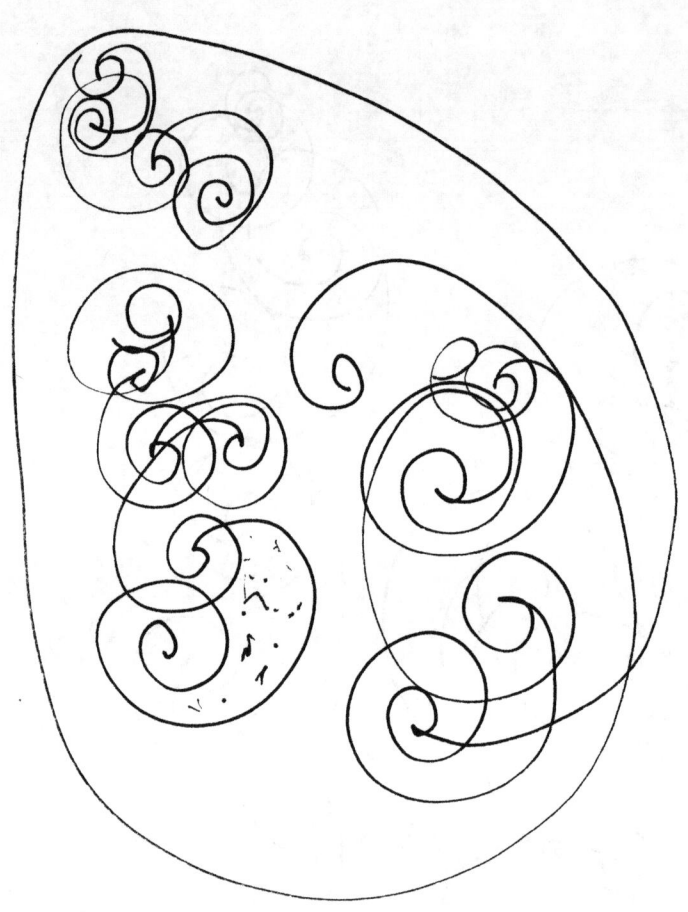

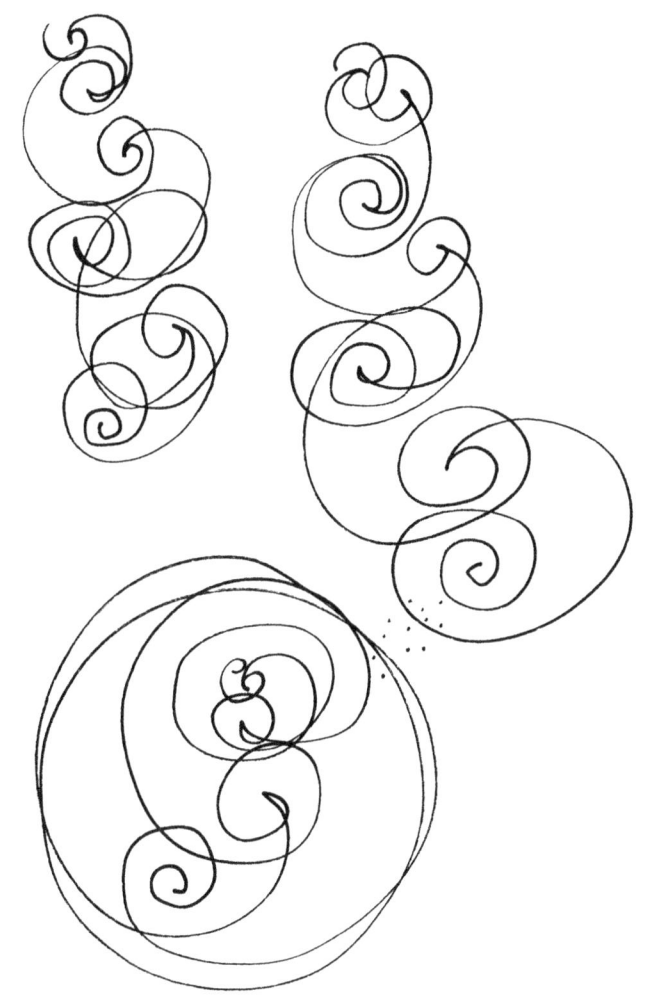

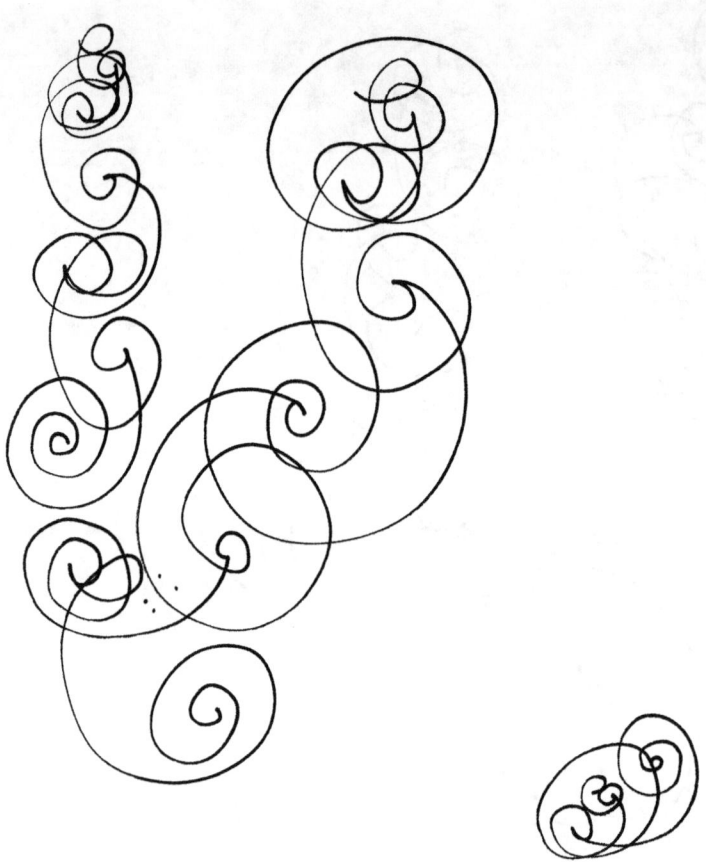

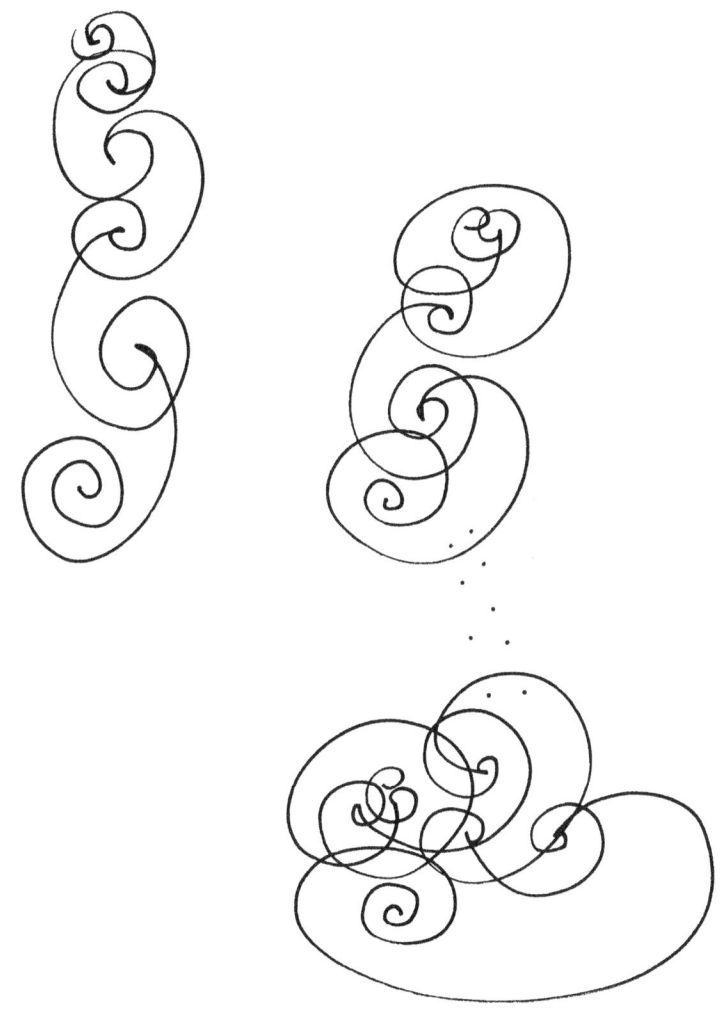

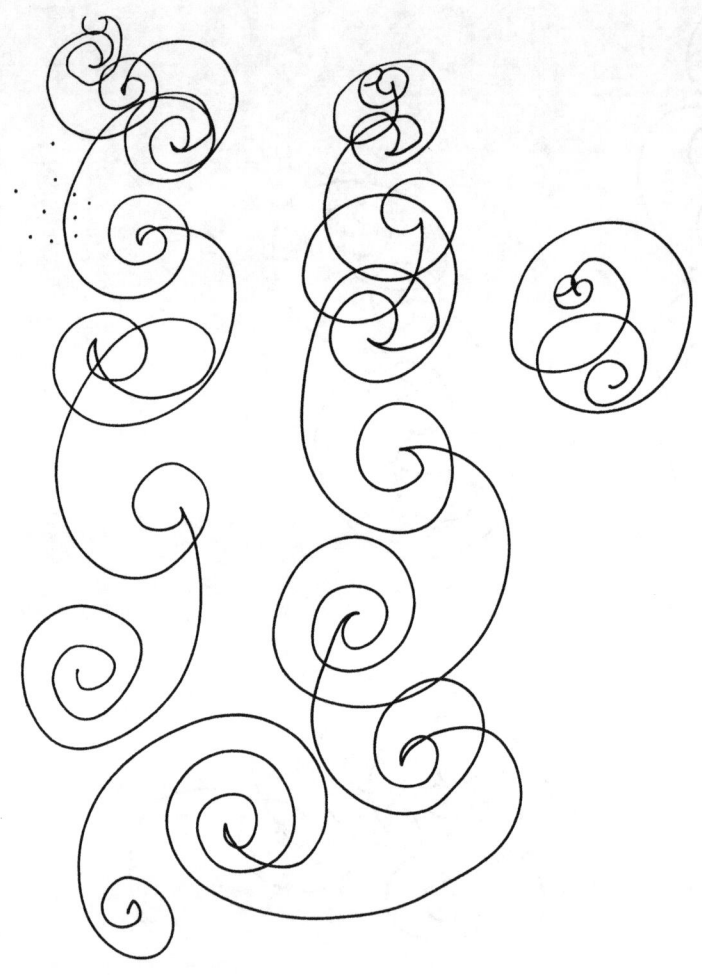

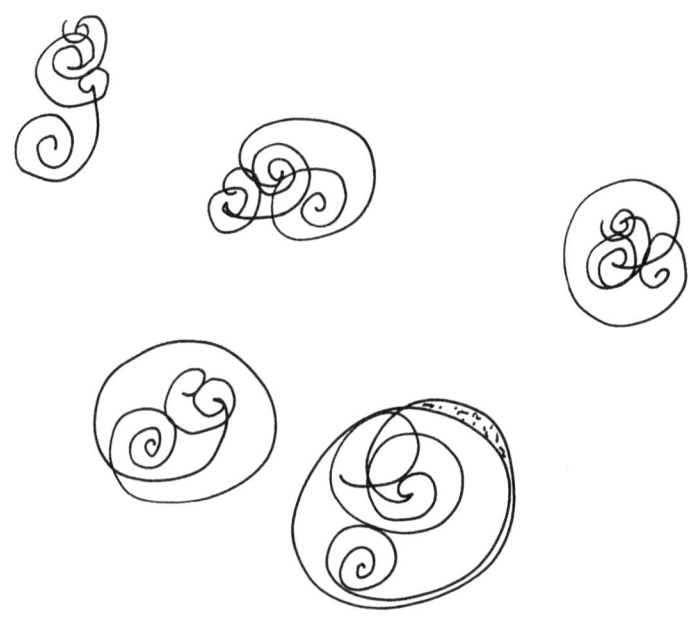

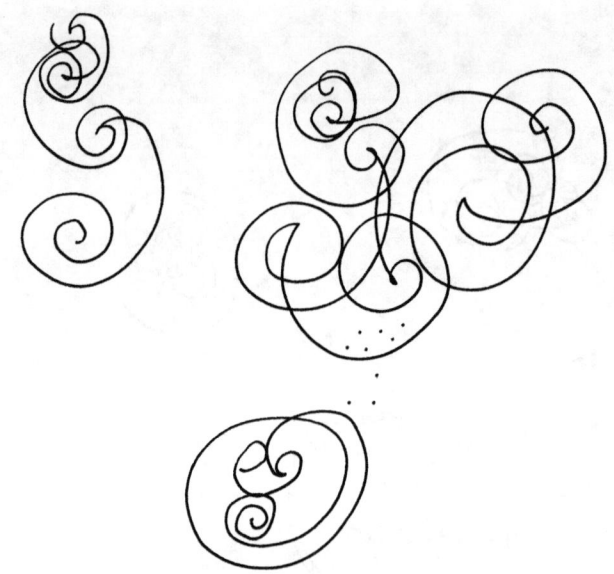

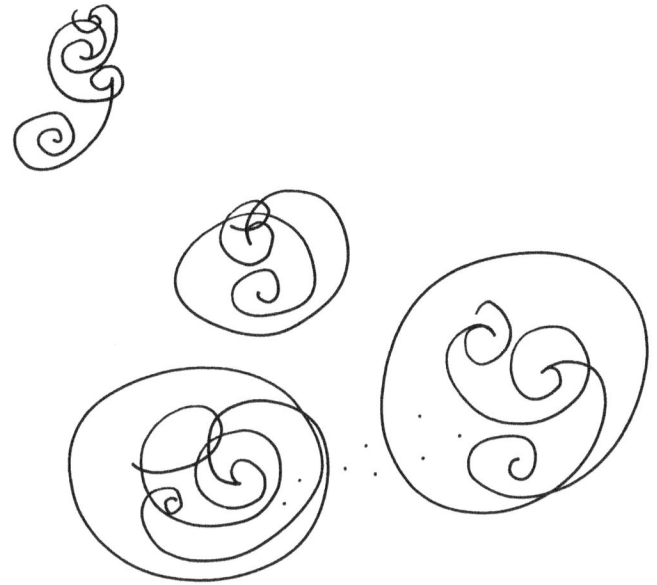

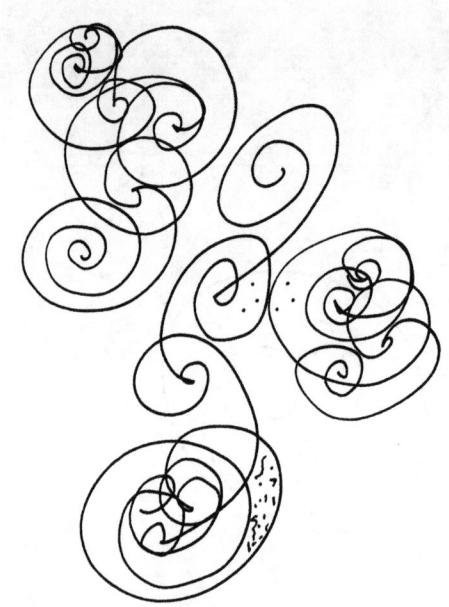

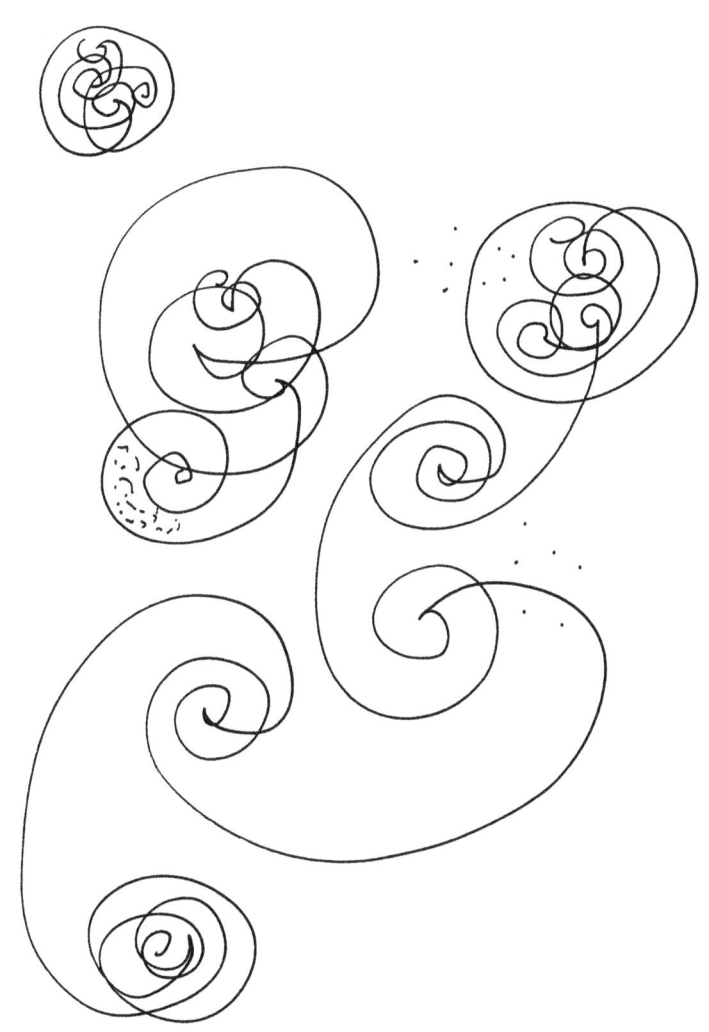

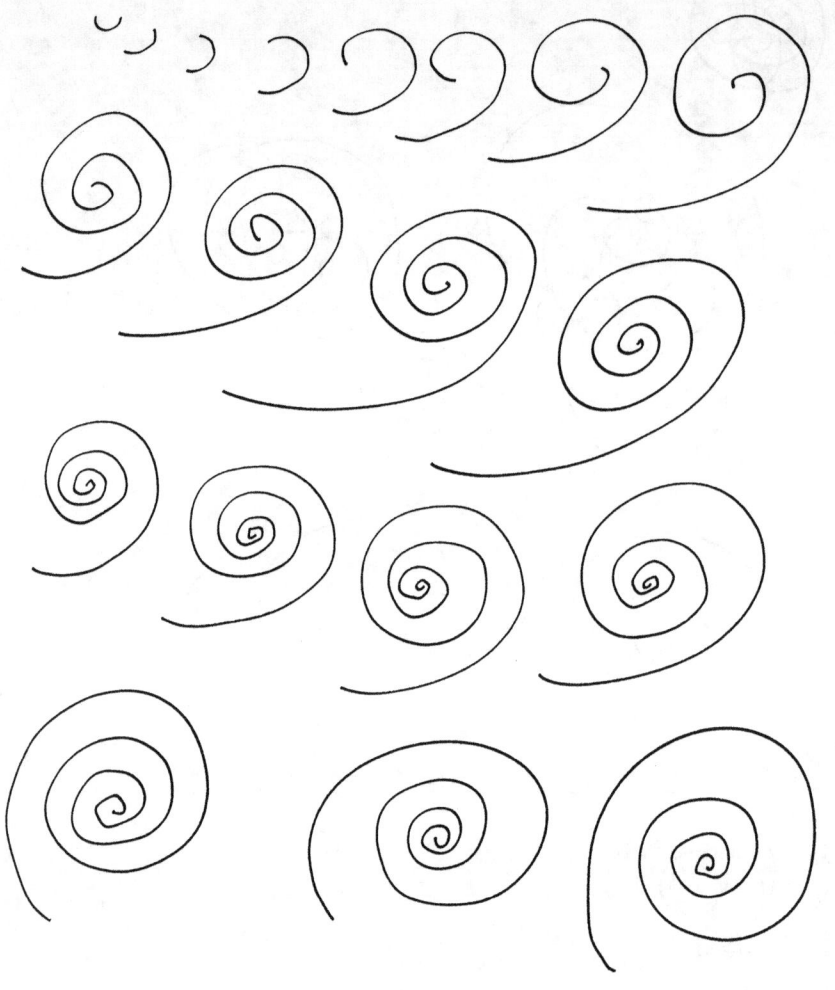

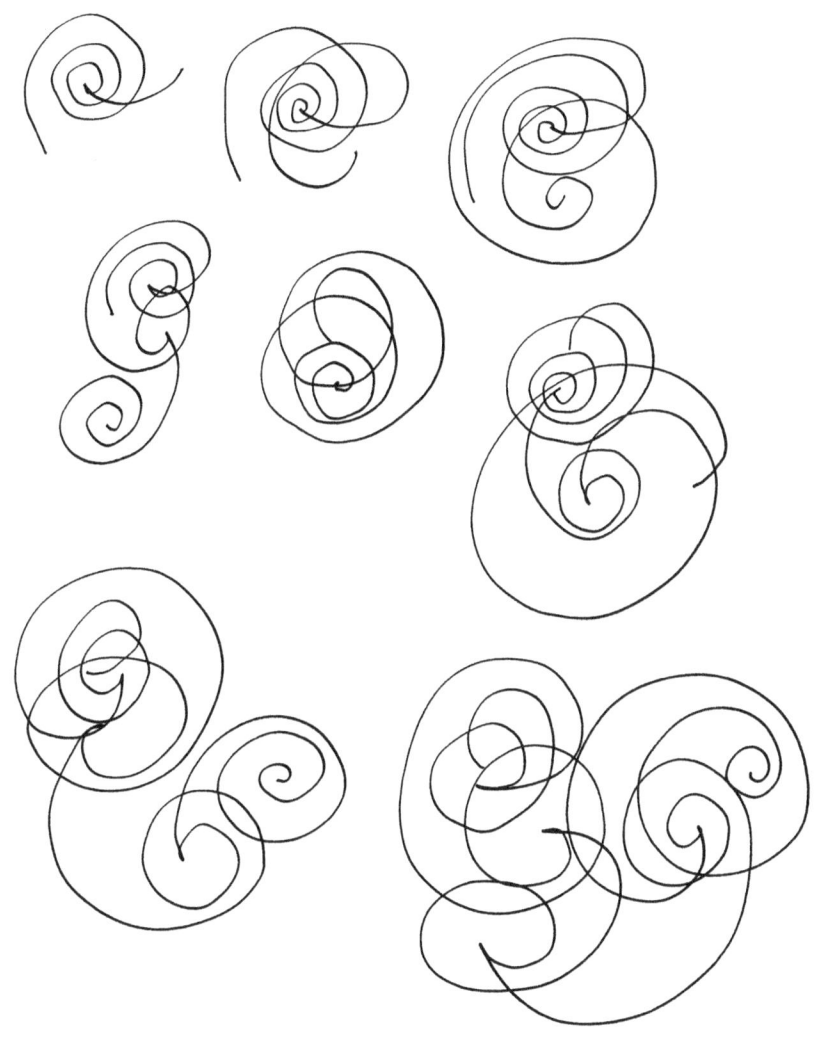

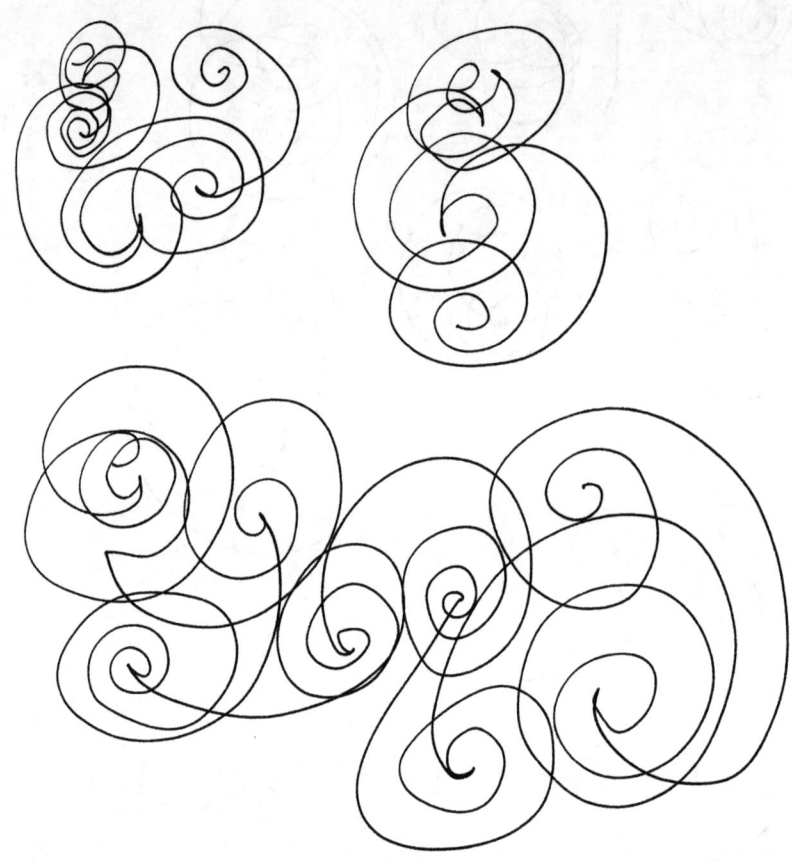

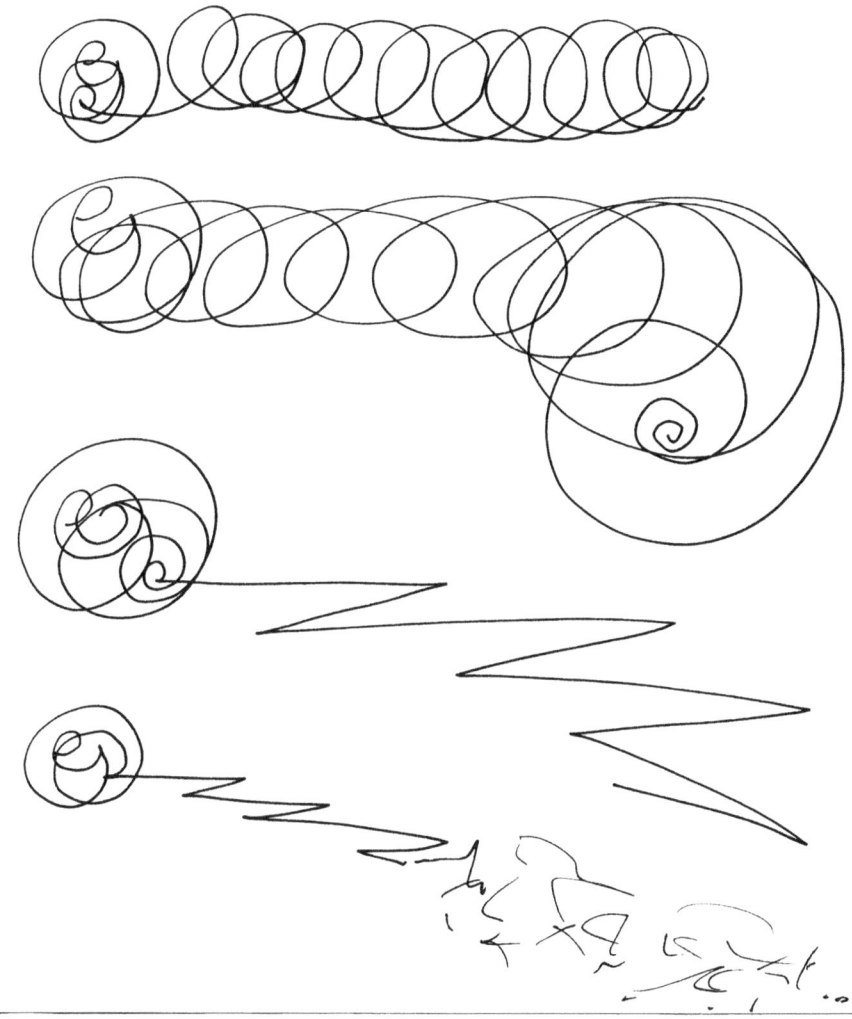

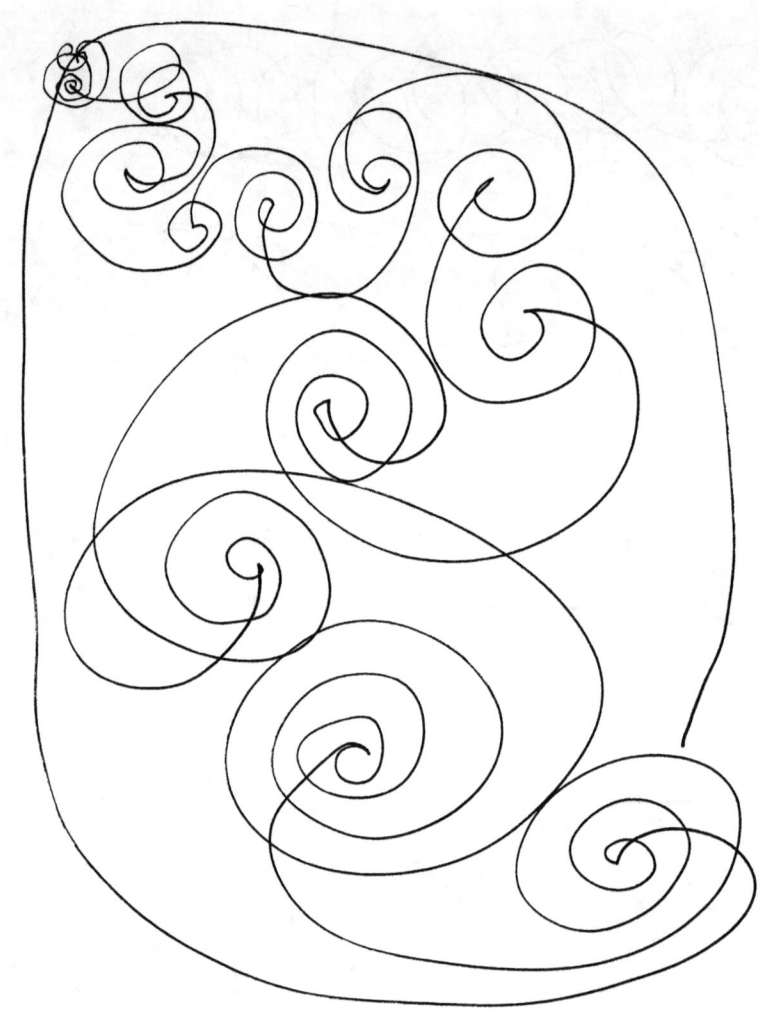

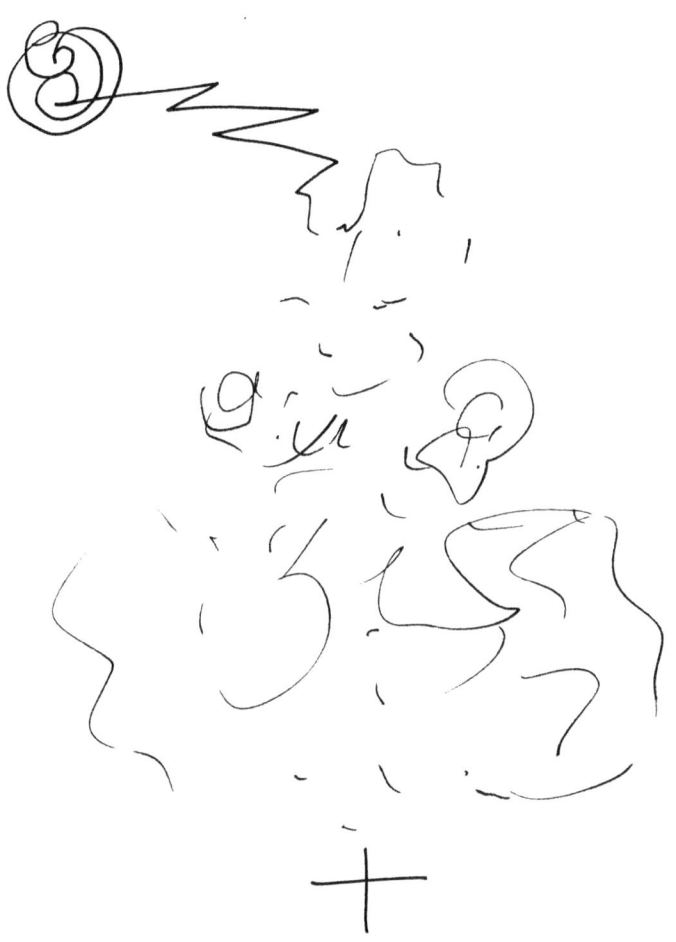

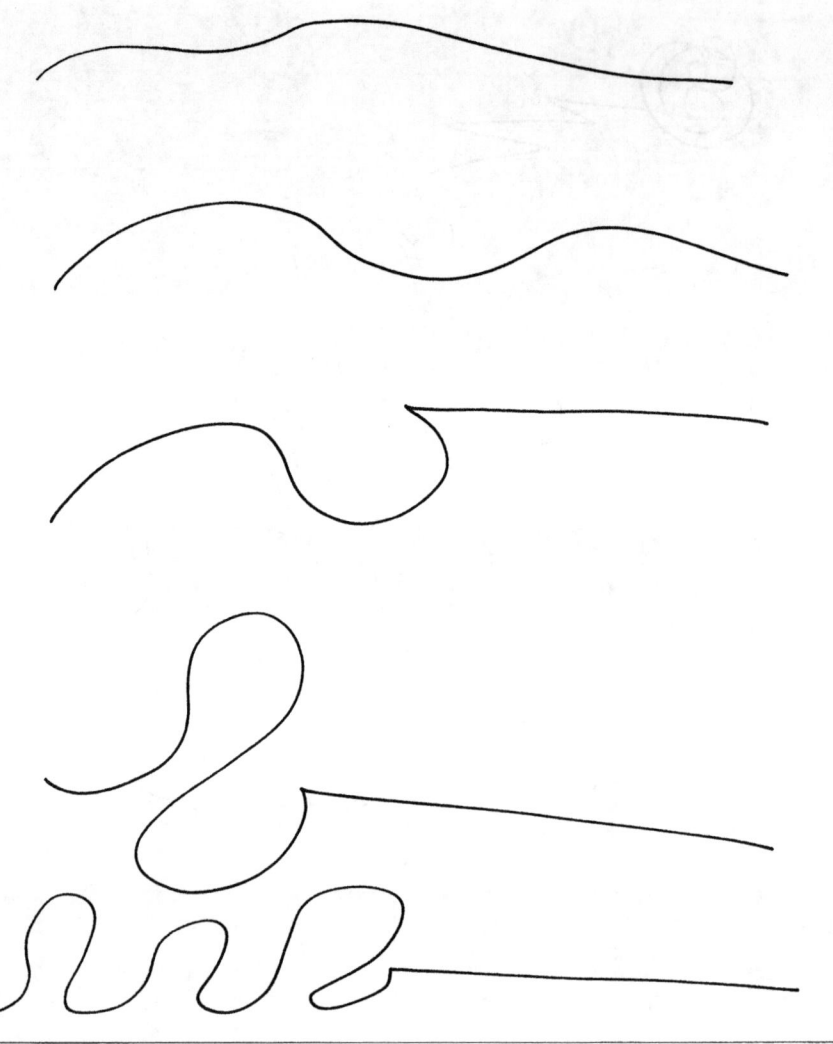

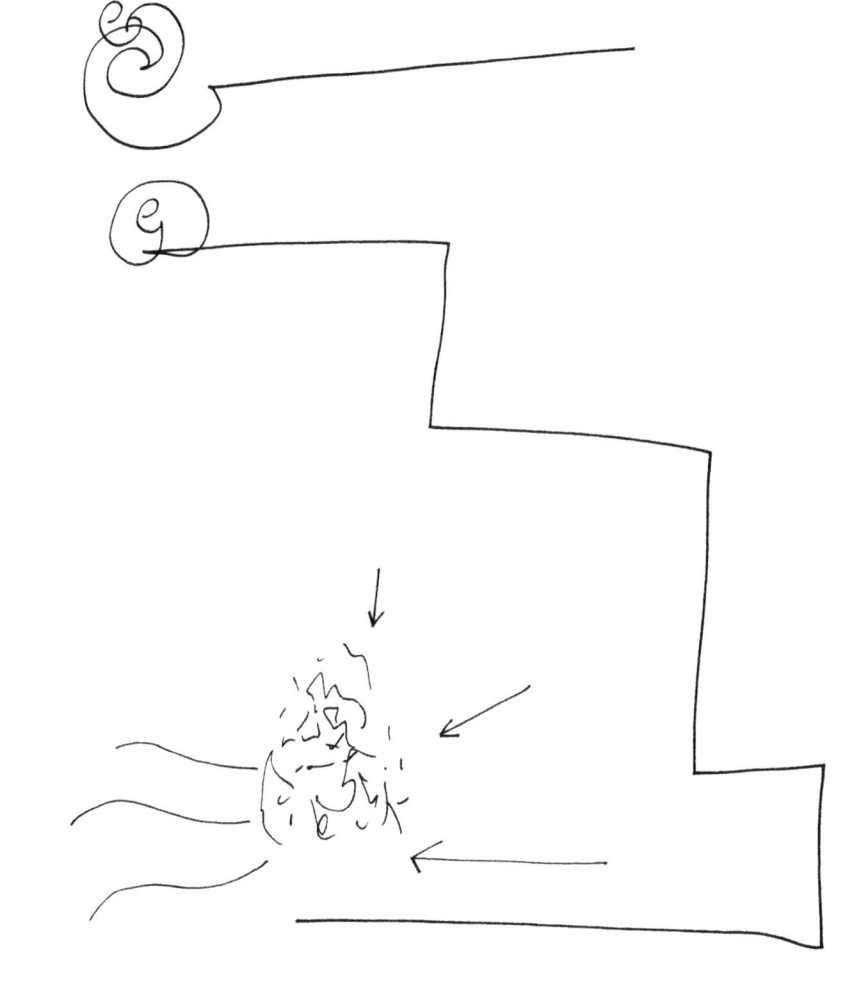

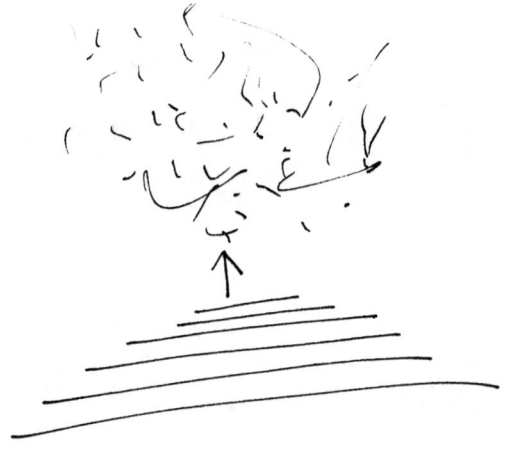

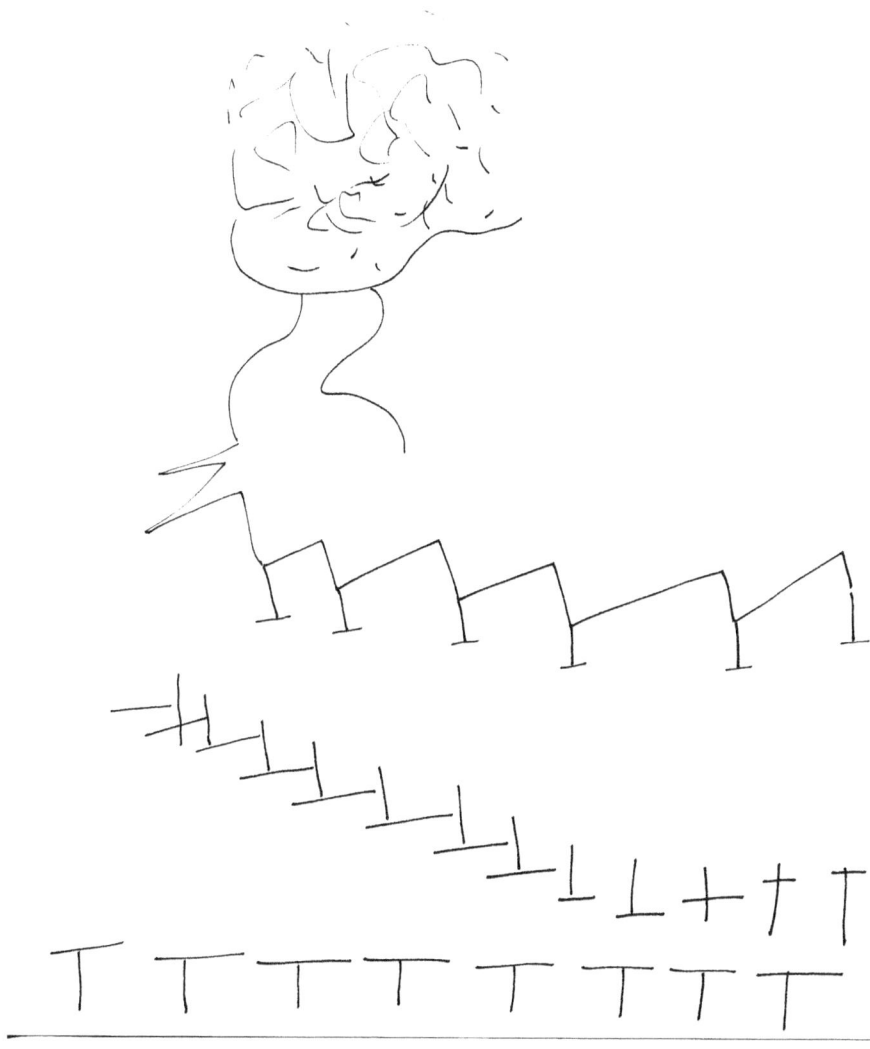

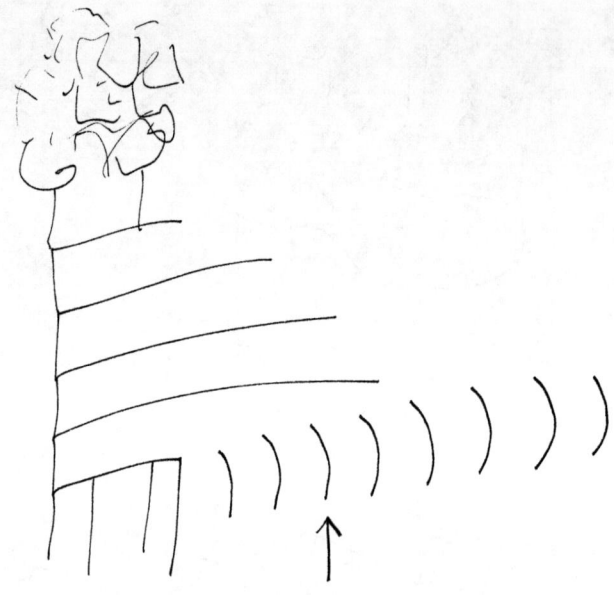

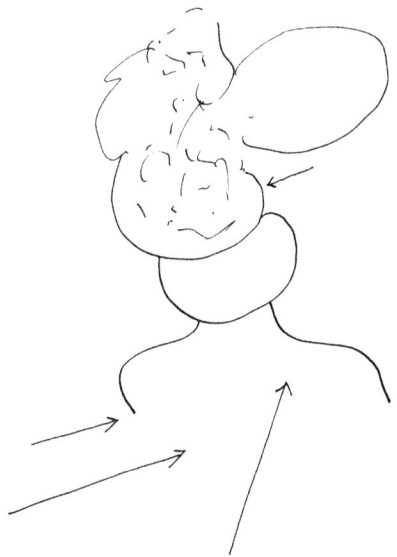

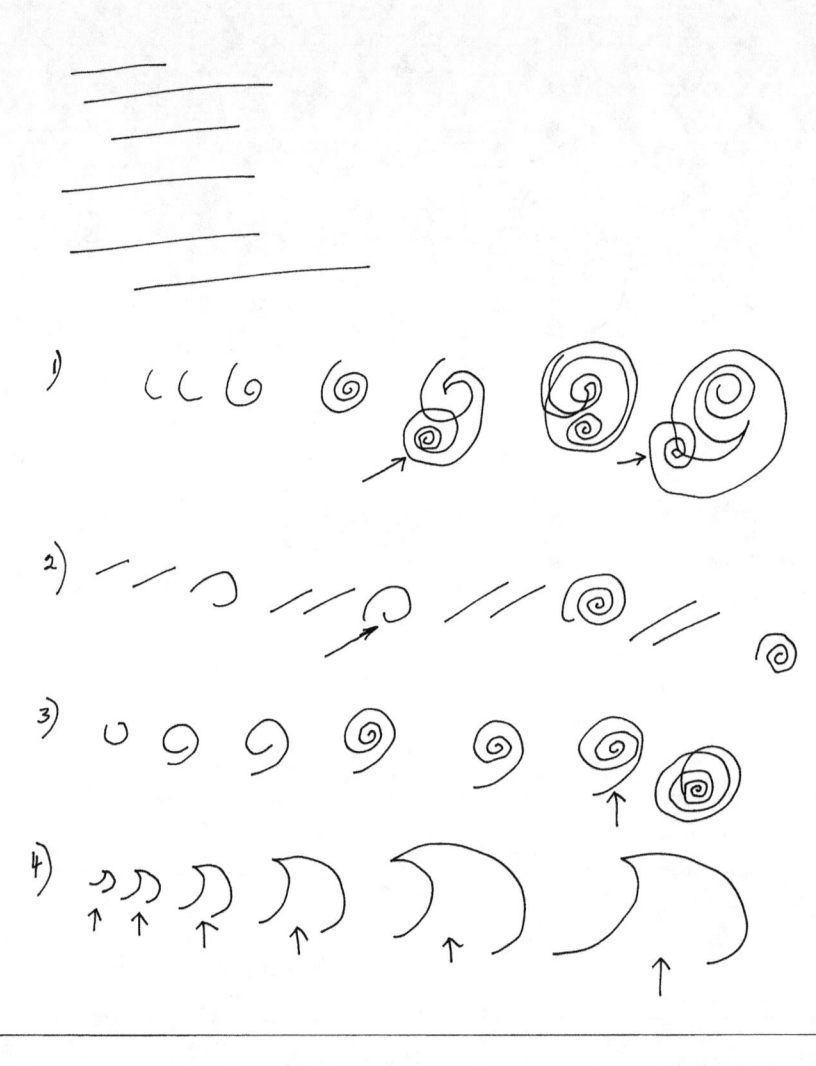

5)

6)

7)

8)

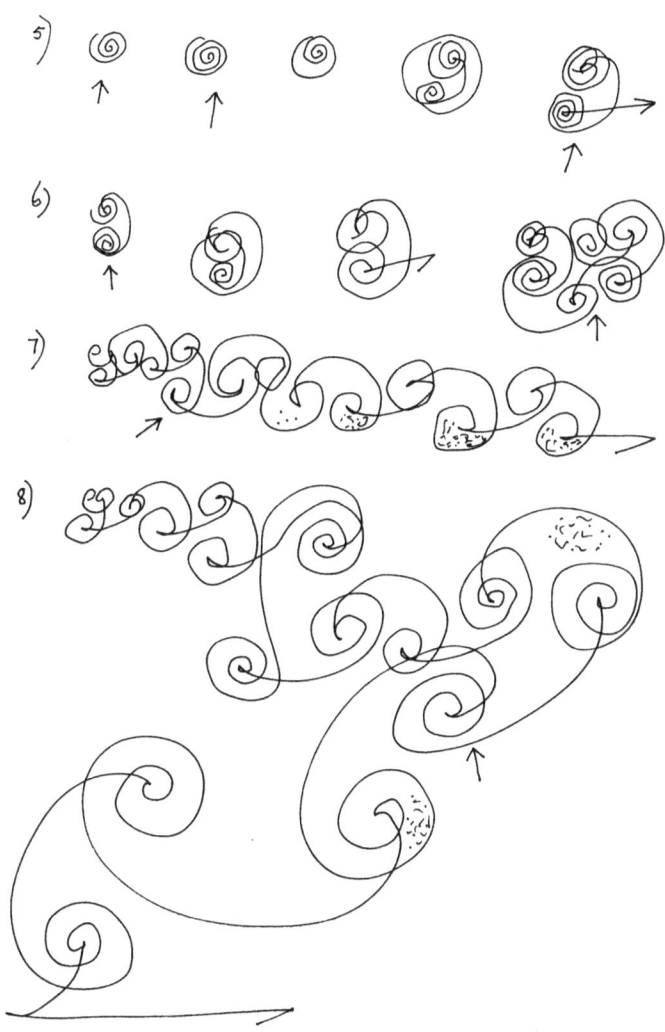

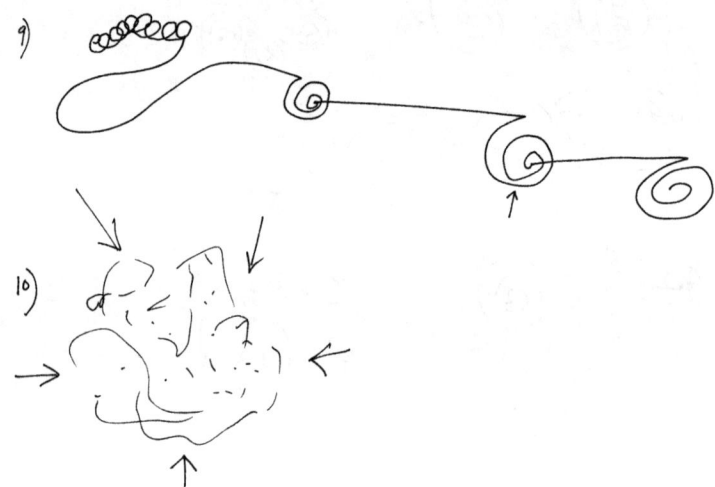

9)

10)

CONTINUED IN VOLUME 6